Occupational therapy and neurological conditions

T0256530

Occupational therapy and neurological conditions

Jenny Preston

Judi Edmans

on behalf of the College of Occupational Therapists Specialist Section – Neurological Practice

WILEY Blackwell

This edition first published 2016 © 2016 by John Wiley & Sons, Ltd

Registered Office
John Wiley & Sons, Ltd, The Atrium, Southern Gate, Chichester, West Sussex, PO19 8SQ, UK

Editorial Offices
9600 Garsington Road, Oxford, OX4 2DQ, UK
The Atrium, Southern Gate, Chichester, West Sussex, PO19 8SQ, UK
111 River Street, Hoboken, NJ 07030-5774, USA

For details of our global editorial offices, for customer services and for information about how to apply for permission to reuse the copyright material in this book please see our website at www.wiley.com/wiley-blackwell

The right of the author to be identified as the author of this work has been asserted in accordance with the UK Copyright, Designs and Patents Act 1988.

All rights reserved. No part of this publication may be reproduced, stored in a retrieval system, or transmitted, in any form or by any means, electronic, mechanical, photocopying, recording or otherwise, except as permitted by the UK Copyright, Designs and Patents Act 1988, without the prior permission of the publisher.

Designations used by companies to distinguish their products are often claimed as trademarks. All brand names and product names used in this book are trade names, service marks, trademarks or registered trademarks of their respective owners. The publisher is not associated with any product or vendor mentioned in this book. It is sold on the understanding that the publisher is not engaged in rendering professional services. If professional advice or other expert assistance is required, the services of a competent professional should be sought.

The contents of this work are intended to further general scientific research, understanding, and discussion only and are not intended and should not be relied upon as recommending or promoting a specific method, diagnosis, or treatment by health science practitioners for any particular patient. The publisher and the author make no representations or warranties with respect to the accuracy or completeness of the contents of this work and specifically disclaim all warranties, including without limitation any implied warranties of fitness for a particular purpose. In view of ongoing research, equipment modifications, changes in governmental regulations, and the constant flow of information relating to the use of medicines, equipment, and devices, the reader is urged to review and evaluate the information provided in the package insert or instructions for each medicine, equipment, or device for, among other things, any changes in the instructions or indication of usage and for added warnings and precautions. Readers should consult with a specialist where appropriate. The fact that an organization or Website is referred to in this work as a citation and/or a potential source of further information does not mean that the author or the publisher endorses the information the organization or Website may provide or recommendations it may make. Further, readers should be aware that Internet Websites listed in this work may have changed or disappeared between when this work was written and when it is read. No warranty may be created or extended by any promotional statements for this work. Neither the publisher nor the author shall be liable for any damages arising herefrom.

Library of Congress Cataloging-in-Publication Data

Names: Edmans, Judi, editor. | Preston, Jenny, 1963– , editor. | College of Occupational Therapists. Specialist Section Neurological Practice, issuing body.
Title: Occupational therapy and neurological conditions / edited by Judi Edmans, Jenny Preston on behalf of the College of Occupational Therapists Specialist Section Neurological Practice.
Description: Chichester, West Sussex ; Hoboken, NJ : John Wiley & Sons, Inc, 2016. |
"This book has been produced by members of the UK College of Occupational Therapists Specialist Section Neurological Practice working with people with long term conditions and has been developed to accompany the 'Occupational therapy and stroke' book." –Preface. | Includes bibliographical references and index.
Identifiers: LCCN 2015047747 (print) | LCCN 2015048300 (ebook) | ISBN 9781118936115 (pbk.) | ISBN 9781118936122 (pdf) | ISBN 9781118936139 (epub)
Subjects: | MESH: Nervous System Diseases–therapy | Occupational Therapy–methods | Case Reports
Classification: LCC RM735 (print) | LCC RM735 (ebook) | NLM WL 140 | DDC 615.8/515–dc23
LC record available at http://lccn.loc.gov/2015047747

A catalogue record for this book is available from the British Library.

Wiley also publishes its books in a variety of electronic formats. Some content that appears in print may not be available in electronic books.

Cover image: [Production Editor to insert]

Set in 9.5/13pt Meridien by SPi Global, Pondicherry, India

Printed in the UK

Contents

List of figures and tables

List of contributors

Ana Aragon   Independent Occupational Therapist, Bath

Catherine Atkinson   Royal Free Neurological Rehabilitation Centre, London

Jill Cooper   Royal Marsden Hospital, London

Jane Duffy   Formerly East Ayrshire Council, now a service user

Judi Edmans   Division of Rehabilitation and Ageing, University of Nottingham, Nottingham

Jo Hurford   National Hospital for Neurology and Neurosurgery, London

Fiona Kelly   Royal Free Neurological Rehabilitation Centre, London

Jill Kings   Neural Pathways, Gateshead, Tyne and Wear

Nicky McNair   Regional Environmental Control Service, North East London Community Services, North East London

Freya Powell   Royal Free Neurological Rehabilitation Centre, London

Jenny Preston   Douglas Grant Rehabilitation Centre, Ayrshire Central Hospital, Irvine

Alison Wiesner   Hertfordshire Neurological Service, Abbotts Langley, Hertfordshire

Academic foreword

Occupational Therapists working with people with neurological conditions will be delighted to learn of the publication of this book. The text has been written by members of the Specialist Section Neurological Practice (UK College of Occupational Therapists) who bring a wealth of knowledge, enthusiasm and clinical expertise to the topic.

Essentially this is a practical guide which provides an excellent reference manual for both those starting out in neurology and for established practitioners. For particular note is the use of case studies which illustrate facts in a way that factual text could not; the account by Jane Duffy of living with HD is particularly moving.

First and foremost this textbook underlines the unique role of occupational therapy in the treatment and care of people with a neurological condition. It incorporates theoretical, clinical and research perspectives to address the impact of neurological conditions from a person-centred viewpoint. The reader should develop an understanding of the impact of managing complex conditions in everyday life.

There are unique skills and contributions occupational therapists can make to improve quality of life in those with neurological conditions. This is an excellent book and I encourage occupational therapists to engage with it and dip into it regularly.

Professor Avril Drummond
Occupational Therapist and Professor of Healthcare Research
University of Nottingham
Nottingham

Service user foreword

It is a pleasure to be asked to write a 'patients view' of this new book regarding the usefulness of input from an occupational therapist with people with a long-term neurological condition. Living with such a condition can lead to many challenges in all aspects of everyday life, social, work and psychological.

This book is focused on assessments of each person as an individual rather than advising the exact same approach and interventions for all patients with a diagnosis; this patient centered approach is one I find reassuring. The emphasis on involving the person in every aspect of decision-making is something that a lot of patients will truly appreciate. To be involved in care decisions is the first step to empowerment for a person suffering from a long-term condition.

Whilst being a book focused on practical work, it pays attention to the importance of evidence-based practice, and the impact the decisions made by the therapist will have on the life of the patient. This offers reassurance to the patient that the interventions will be safe, effective and proved to have worked elsewhere.

As a layperson reading this it offers some enlightenment to the true meaning of occupation and the multiple facets of this rather than it just being simply about remaining at work through an illness. The interventions a therapist can use in all areas of a patient's life become more valuable as each patient's needs are different. I hope new and experienced therapists alike will find this book helpful in their ongoing learning and development as professionals and therefore more patients will benefit from the subsequent input from the therapists.

Tony Wilde
Service User
Nottingham

Preface

This book has been produced by members of the UK College of Occupational Therapists Specialist Section – Neurological Practice working with people with long-term conditions and has been developed to accompany the book titled *Occupational Therapy and Stroke*.

The book is intended for use by newly qualified occupational therapists and those new to the field of the management of people with long-term neurological conditions. It acknowledges 'occupation' as the foundation of occupational therapy, explaining how this combined with our core skills facilitates an understanding of the complexities of occupational therapy clinical practice with people with long-term neurological conditions.

We have tried to offer a guide from theory to clinical practice basing this around the four most common long-term neurological conditions: Huntington's disease (HD), motor neurone disease (MND), multiple sclerosis (MS) and Parkinson's. We hope that by providing guidance and explanations, new graduates will feel confident in the management of people with long-term neurological conditions.

Throughout the book we have included client quotes and case studies to provide real-life presentations to put the theory into context.

For ease of terminology throughout this book, the 'client/patient' is referred to as 'the client' where it is in reference to our own work, irrespective of whether he/she is being treated in the hospital or community. However, the term 'patient' is left unchanged where it is in reference to a national project/referenced document, etc. Similarly, we have used the term 'Parkinson's' throughout this book, as this is currently the correct term for the condition previously known as 'Parkinson's disease'.

In the future, as new ideas are developed, this text should be viewed in the light of developing practice.

Dr Judi Edmans
Co-Editor

Acknowledgements

We would like to give particular thanks to Dr Avril Drummond for providing Academic Foreword; Tony Wilde for providing Service User Foreword; all the contributors for their contributions; all those providing permission for the inclusion of photographs, figures and tables; the College of Occupational Therapists Specialist Section – Neurological Practice for funding to enable us to prepare this book; and last but not least our long-suffering husbands and families for their endless support and patience during the time taken to prepare this book.

Dr Jenny Preston and Dr Judi Edmans
Co-Editors

CHAPTER 1

Introduction

1.1 Economic impact of long-term neurological conditions

It is estimated that 10 million people in the United Kingdom live with some form of neurological condition that impacts on their everyday lives (Department of Health [DoH], 2005). Neurological conditions account for one in five emergency hospital admissions, one in eight general practice consultations and a high proportion of severe and progressive disability in the population (Association of British Neurologists, 2003). As many as 350 000 people in the United Kingdom need help with activities of daily living because of a neurological condition and 850 000 people care for someone with a neurological condition (DoH, 2005). Due to their devastating impact and their generally progressive nature, neurological conditions are considered as long-term affecting individuals throughout their life span.

Occupational therapy is defined as 'a client-centred health profession concerned with promoting health and well-being through occupation enabling people to participate in everyday life' (World Federation of Occupational Therapists, 2011). Occupational therapy practice focuses on enabling individuals to modify and adapt elements of their roles, occupations or environments to support occupational participation in response to changes within their lives. Occupational therapists have a key role to play in supporting people living with a long-term neurological condition to manage a life of unpredictability and uncertainty. This requires a complex combination of knowledge and skills to address the physical, psychological, cognitive and emotional needs of people together with a broad range of assessments and interventions.

Occupational Therapy and Neurological Conditions, First Edition. Edited by Jenny Preston and Judi Edmans.
© 2016 John Wiley & Sons, Ltd. Published 2016 by John Wiley & Sons, Ltd.

1.2 Definition of long-term neurological conditions

The DoH (2005) describes 'long-term neurological conditions' as

a range of conditions affecting the brain or spinal cord which occur through a variety of mechanisms which include the following:
- Sudden onset conditions (e.g. acquired brain injury of any cause, stroke and spinal cord injury)
- Intermittent conditions (e.g. epilepsy)
- Progressive conditions (e.g. multiple sclerosis (MS), motor neurone disease (MND), Parkinson's and other degenerative disorders)
- Stable conditions with/without age-related degeneration (e.g. polio or cerebral palsy).

This book specifically focuses on the following progressive neurological conditions:
- Huntington's disease (HD)
- Motor neurone disease (MND)
- Multiple sclerosis (MS)
- Parkinson's.

  Whilst there is an abundance of literature relating to each of these medical conditions the primary aim of this book is to place this knowledge and understanding within the context of occupational therapy practice. In order to fully understand the holistic needs of their clients occupational therapists are required to develop knowledge of the underlying pathology of each of these neurological conditions. However this understanding from a medical perspective should not be assumed to represent a medical model of care with an emphasis on symptomatic management. Throughout this book the focus is on delivering person-centred models of practice which support the complexity of the needs of people with neurological conditions from an occupational perspective.

1.3 International Classification of Functioning, Disability and Health

The International Classification of Functioning, Disability and Health (ICF) offers a conceptual basis for the definition and measurement of health and disability (World Health Organisation [WHO], 2002). Developed within a biopsychosocial model, ICF views disability and functioning as outcomes of interactions between **health conditions** (diseases, disorders and injuries) and **contextual factors**, as shown in Figure 1.1. Amongst contextual factors are external environmental factors (e.g., social attitudes, architectural characteristics, legal and social structures) and internal factors which include gender, age, coping styles, social background,

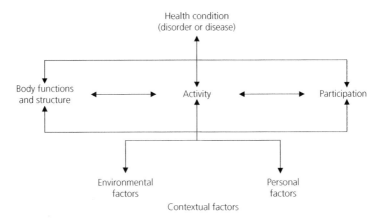

Figure 1.1 Model of disability that is the basis for ICF. (Source: WHO, 2002, p. 9. Reproduced with permission of World Health Organisation.)

Box 1.1 Formal definitions of the components of ICF.

Body functions are physiological functions of body systems (including psychological functions).
Body structures are anatomical parts of the body such as organs, limbs and their components.
Impairments are problems in body function or structure such as significant deviation or loss.
Activity is the execution of a task or action by an individual.
Participation is involvement in a life situation.
Activity limitations are difficulties an individual may experience in involvement in life situations.
Participation restrictions are problems an individual may experience in involvement in life situations.
Environmental factors make up the physical, social and attitudinal environment in which people live and conduct their lives.

Source: WHO (2002, p. 10). Reproduced with permission of World Health Organisation.

past and current experience, character and other factors that influence how disability is experienced by the individual (WHO, 2002).

Within this framework ICF defines three levels of human functioning: functioning at the level of body or body part (**impairment**), the whole person (**activity limitations**) and the whole person in a social context (**participation restrictions**). The formal definitions of these components of ICF are provided in Box 1.1 (WHO, 2002).

The remainder of this chapter presents each of the four neurological conditions in relation to body functions, body structures and impairments, highlighting the differences and similarities of each condition. Subsequent chapters explore the wider implications for activity and participation.

1.4 Huntington's disease

HD is a rare disease, affecting an estimated 7–10 people per 100 000 or somewhere in the region of between 4200 and 6000 people in the United Kingdom (Quarrell, 2008). The onset of the disease is insidious and the age of onset depends on a number of different factors. Most people develop the condition between the ages of 30 and 50 years, but the disease can appear in all age groups (Nance et al., 2013). The HD gene is dominant, which means that each child of a parent with HD has a 50% chance of inheriting the disease and is said to be 'at-risk'. Males and females have the same risk of inheriting the disease. HD occurs in all races (Nance et al., 2013).

There is currently no cure or treatment which can halt, slow or reverse the progression of the disease (Nance et al., 2013) and people with HD tend to die, on average, between 15 and 16 years after the onset of symptoms (Quarrell, 2008). People don't die from HD itself, but they die from complications such as choking, heart failure, and infection or aspiration pneumonia (Nance et al., 2013).

1.4.1 Body functions
HD is a hereditary neurodegenerative genetic disorder caused by an expansion of a repeating CAG triplet series in the huntingtin gene on chromosome 4, which results in a protein with an abnormally long polyglutamine sequence (Nance et al., 2013).

1.4.2 Body structures
HD causes cells in the brain to die, specifically the caudate and the putamen and, as the disease progresses, the cerebral cortex. These organic changes lead to cognitive, motor and psychiatric changes that have a devastating impact on the individual. As the brain cells die, a person with HD becomes less able to control their movements, recall events, make decisions and control their emotions (Nance et al., 2013).

1.4.3 Stages of HD
Early stage
Symptoms may include minor involuntary movements, subtle loss of coordination, difficulty thinking through complex problems, depression, irritability, or disinhibition (Nance et al., 2013). Early symptoms of the disease often include subtle cognitive changes including the following:
• Difficulty organising routine matters or coping effectively with new situations
• Difficulty recalling information may make them appear forgetful
• Work activities may become more time-consuming
• Decision-making and attention to details may be impaired
• Irritability

- Slight physical changes may also develop at this stage. There can be involuntary movements which may initially consist of 'nervous' activity, fidgeting, a twitching of the hands or feet, or excessive restlessness. Individuals may also notice a little awkwardness, changes in handwriting or difficulty with daily tasks such as driving (Nance et al., 2013).

Middle stage

Chorea may be prominent, and people with HD have increasing difficulty with voluntary motor tasks. There may be issues with swallowing, balance, falls and weight loss. Problem solving becomes more difficult due to difficulties sequencing, organising or prioritising information (Nance et al., 2013).

The initial physical symptoms will gradually develop into more obvious involuntary movements such as jerking and twitching of the head, neck and arms and legs. These movements may interfere with walking, speaking and swallowing. People at this stage of HD often stagger when they walk and their speech may become slurred. They may have increasing difficulty working or managing a household, but they can still deal with most activities of daily living (Nance et al., 2013).

Late stage

Chorea may be severe, or be replaced by rigidity, dystonia and bradykinesia. Although they are unable to speak in the end stages, it is important to note that people with HD retain a level of comprehension (Nance et al., 2013). People in these stages of HD can no longer manage the activities of daily living and usually require professional nursing care. Difficulties with swallowing and weight loss are common (Nance et al., 2013).

1.4.4 Impairments

- Chorea
  More than 90% of people with HD have chorea. It is characterised by 'involuntary movements which are often sudden, irregular and purposeless or semi-purposeless. The movements are often more prominent in the extremities early in the disease, but progress to include facial grimacing, eyelid elevation, neck, shoulder, trunk, and leg movements as the disease progresses' (Nance et al., 2013).
- Dystonia
  Characterised by 'a repetitive, abnormal pattern of muscle contraction which is frequently associated with a twisting quality' (Nance et al., 2013).
- Bradykinesia
  'Slowness of movement can include loss of facial expressivity, absence of arm swing, rapid alternating movements and gait slowness' (Nance et al., 2013).
- Tics
  'are sudden brief, intermittent movements, gestures or vocalisations which can occur with HD. Respiratory and vocal tics can produce sniffs, grunts, moans or coughs' (Nance et al., 2013).

- Loss of motor control
  - Progressive loss of voluntary motor control
  - Clumsy, awkward movement
  - Akinetic
  - Rigidity
  - Hyper reflexia
  - Extensor plantar reflexes (Nance et al., 2013)
- Gait impairment and falls
  - Slower wide-based gait
  - Trunk dystonia
  - Chorea
  - Displaced centre of gravity (Nance et al., 2013)
- Communication and swallowing
  - Dysarthria
  - Changes in speech rhythm
  - Voice changes, that is soft spoken or explosive
  - Complete loss of speech often occurs
  - Difficulties with speech initiation
  - Word-finding difficulties
  - Impaired breathing (Nance et al., 2013)
  - Dysphagia
  - Aspiration
- Bowel and bladder dysfunction
- Weight Loss
- Cognitive impairment
  - Attentional deficits
  - Speed of processing
  - Memory
  - Visuospatial abilities
  - Executive function
  - Planning
  - Lack of insight
  - Behavioural regulation
  - Lack of initiation
  - Perseveration
  - Impulse control (Huntington's Disease Association, 2012)
- Emotional and behavioural changes
  - Depression
  - Apathy
  - Irritability
  - Disinhibition
  - Jocularity

- Obsessive compulsive disorder
- Impaired judgement
- Mania
- Agitation
- Delirium
- Sexual disorders including loss of libido or making inappropriate sexual demands (Huntington's Disease Association, 2012)

1.4.5 Diagnosing HD

Genetic testing in HD can serve two purposes: as a diagnostic tool and as a predictive test to identify level of risk. Genetic testing involves the examination of an individual's DNA, which is obtained from a blood sample. DNA molecules consist of four bases, known as A (adenine), T (thymine), G (guanine) and C (cytosine). The gene that causes HD is called the HD gene, and within it there is a region in which a sequence of the three bases (CAG) is repeated many times. For individuals with HD, the CAG sequence has increased (expanded) into a range that is abnormal. Testing is done in a specialised laboratory to determine the number of CAG repeats in both copies of the HD gene (Huntington's Disease Association, 2012).

An HD gene expansion is passed on in families and children of a parent with this expansion have a 50% chance of developing the disease. Predictive testing is a process whereby an individual at risk of the disease can discover whether or not they have inherited the expanded HD gene, and will go on to develop HD. A 'gene negative' result is where the number of CAG repeats is 26 or less. The individual will not go on to develop the HD and their children will not be at increased risk either (Huntington's Disease Association, 2012).

An intermediate result is a result where the number of CAG repeats is between 27 and 35. This means that the individual will not go on to develop HD but, in some cases, may pass on an expansion to their children because the CAG repeat can be unstable when passed from one generation to the next. This can mean that sometimes children will be at higher risk for developing HD (Huntington's Disease Association, 2012).

A reduced penetrance result is one where the number of CAG repeats is between 36 and 39. An individual with a result in this range may not develop any symptoms of HD; however, this result also means that the next generation may be at risk of inheriting a larger expansion as it would also be unstable (Huntington's Disease Association, 2012).

A full penetrance or 'gene positive' is a result where the number of CAG repeats is 40 or more. The individual with this result will always go on to develop HD at some point in the future. The result does not give information on the age of onset of symptoms (Huntington's Disease Association, 2012).

Case study

Luke is 41 years old. Last year Luke underwent genetic testing following the death of his father to Huntington's disease 8 years ago. Although Luke was aware of the genetic risk of HD he previously did not feel able to cope with genetic testing and opted to continue life without knowing the potential risk. However as he began to realise that some potential signs might be emerging within his everyday life, he felt it was now necessary for him to have a more definite prediction of what might lie ahead. It was confirmed that Luke had a full penetrance result confirming that he would go on to develop HD. Luke was devastated by the outcome as he now had two young children of his own. While Luke had been aware of his father's condition he previously refused to attend for genetic counselling. Luke and his wife Amy aspired to have a normal family life and did not wish to acknowledge the potential risks when planning their family.

Luke works as a self-employed plumbing and heating engineer. Recently he had noticed some slight clumsiness or lack of co-ordination when working with his tools. This did not really impact on his ability to complete jobs, but he found he was becoming slightly weaker when unscrewing tight fastenings, greater difficulty when working within confined spaces and some difficulties with tasks requiring the simultaneous use of both hands. He was aware that it was taking him longer to complete jobs which placed him under significant pressure as in his trade time was money and this could have significant financial implications if he was unable to accept the same number of jobs. He also had many regular customers and had spent several years building a reputation as a reliable and dependable tradesman. Luke did not wish to let his customers down.

In addition to the practical aspects of his job Luke was also aware that he was finding it harder to plan his work schedule. He felt he was wasting valuable time as he was not planning his jobs in the same way to minimise travel time, and on occasions was significantly under-estimating how long it would take to complete a job. Previously Luke would have done this automatically, but now he was finding that he had to give this much more thought and was becoming angry and frustrated with himself because of this. There had also been some occasions when Luke had turned up for a job but had not brought the right tools or equipment. Again this had time and financial implications for him.

Luke also had responsibility for the administration aspects of his business including tax returns, book-keeping, preparation of customer invoices, and he was very concerned that he was making some mistakes with this. Luke had previously been a bit of a perfectionist, but now he was regularly making small mistakes and errors. Initially he attributed this to tiredness as he worked long hours, but he didn't cope well with this change and got very frustrated with himself for making mistakes. He was starting to doubt his own ability and found himself taking more time to check his work to see that it was accurate.

Amy was aware of changes in Luke as he was forgetting things that she had told him during conversations. There were numerous occasions when Luke would say 'You never told me that...' when Amy was confident that a discussion had taken place. Luke had previously been very gentle and mild mannered and loved spending time with his family. More recently Luke had become irritable with Amy and the children. He seemed less tolerant of the children's behaviour and seemed to be more reactive and angry with them all.

On occasions Luke had made rather unusual comments to people such as when waiting in the queue in the supermarket, or when trying to find a parking space. Amy was quite embarrassed by this and was concerned that Luke did not seem to understand why this might be inappropriate. Luke was very aware of twitching in his hands and feet and was quite uncomfortable about this when he was out in public. Amy felt that some of Luke's seemingly inappropriate comments to people were due to the fact that Luke thought they were staring at him.

Although Amy and Luke felt they were coping well with the diagnosis, it was clear that they were not able to talk to each other about their worries, concerns, hopes and wishes. This was contributing to pressures within their relationship and both were becoming very low in mood. The HD Specialist Nurse was involved in Luke's care and recognised the need for practical support for Luke and his family and initiated a referral to occupational therapy.

Luke initially refused to be referred to an occupational therapist but in time rather reluctantly agreed to this. It quickly became apparent that Luke's attitude was that 'nothing could be done to make him better', that he 'had created this problem for his children' and that 'he was responsible for their future', including the potential risk of their development of HD. Luke felt he was letting everybody around him down as his family relied on him for financial support and that he should be providing for his family. Luke worried for Amy and the potential that she might need to care for him as the disease progressed. He did not feel that Amy was strong enough to cope with this as she had experienced problems with depression in the past following the birth of their children. Luke did not wish to burden his mother who was still working through the loss of his father.

1.5 Motor neurone disease

MND is a term used to describe a group of related diseases that attack the motor neurones (MND Association, 2012). It is a life-limiting condition that progressively impacts on the ability to perform daily functions. The average age at symptom onset is between 50 and 70 years, although it may occur earlier or later in life. Typically symptoms such as stumbling, foot drop, weakened grip, slurred speech, cramp, muscle wasting and fatigue occur in the early stages becoming progressively worse over a 2–5-year period. The current incidence is $2:100000$ per annum, rising with age and prevalence rates of $7:100000$, with a male:female ratio of $3:2$ (MND Association, 2012).

Amyotrophic lateral sclerosis
Around 85% of people with MND will be diagnosed with amyotrophic lateral sclerosis (ALS). Early symptoms can include muscle weakness with spasticity in the upper or lower limbs which become progressively worse over a 2–5-year period. Where the initial onset is in the bulbar territory, survival tends to be shorter (2–3 years) (MND Association, 2012).

Progressive bulbar palsy
In this form of MND early bulbar signs can be relatively confined for several months before limb involvement becomes apparent. The overall survival rate for this form is 6 months to 4 years with a gender ratio of $1:3$ male:female (MND Association, 2012).

Progressive muscular atrophy

Affecting less than 10% of people with MND progressive muscular atrophy (PMA) is characterised by a slowly progressive, proximal upper limb weakness which is usually symmetrical, and accompanied by visible fasciculations (MND Association, 2012).

Primary lateral sclerosis

This is the rarest form affecting approximately 5% of people with MND. It is characterised by spasticity and increased reflex response, as only upper motor neurone damage occurs. Often balance is affected and survival is notably longer (10–20 years) (MND Association, 2012).

1.5.1 Body functions

The motor neurone diseases are a group of progressive neurological disorders that destroy motor neurones, the cells that control essential voluntary muscle activity such as speaking, walking, breathing and swallowing.

1.5.2 Body structures

Motor neurones are nerve cells which carry an electrical transmission from the central nervous system to the muscles triggering a muscle to either contract or relax. The damage which occurs in MND leads to an interruption in the electrical transmission, resulting in a breakdown in the communications between the brain and the muscles. Impairment of the upper motor neurones leads to weakness and stiffness in the muscles, while lower motor neurone damage results in weak, floppy muscles and fasciculations (MND Association, 2013; Figure 1.2).

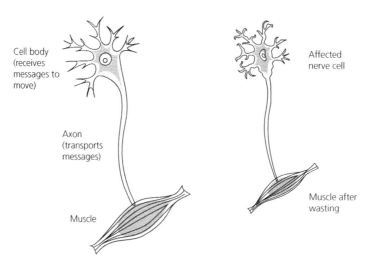

Cell body (receives messages to move)

Axon (transports messages)

Muscle

Affected nerve cell

Muscle after wasting

Figure 1.2 Comparison of healthy and motor neurone affected by MND. (Source: MND Association, 2013, p. 7. Reproduced with permission of MND Association.)

1.5.3 Genetic Risk
Sporadic MND
While there is no known reason currently why some people may be at greater risk than others of developing MND genetic susceptibility and environmental factors may contribute to increased chance. For 90–95% of people diagnosed with MND, there is no family history of the disease (MND Association, 2012).

Familial MND
Of the remaining 5–10%, however, the disease is caused by genetic mutation. Currently there is no genetic test available that can confirm whether or not the disease is familial. Familial MND nearly always displays autosomal dominant inheritance, although penetrance is sometimes reduced, and the disease can appear to skip a generation. Age and site of onset can vary between cases within the same family (MND Association, 2012).

1.5.4 Impairments
- Muscle weakness
- Spasticity or stiffness in the limb muscles
- Slow and effortful movements
- Knee and ankle jerks
- Sudden muscle cramps
- Loss of voluntary movement
- Twitching and fasciculation
- Pain
- Dysarthria
- Dysphagia
- Respiratory insufficiency
- Acute dyspnoea
- Saliva and mucus problems
- Fatigue
- Constipation
- Cognitive changes including executive functions and memory problems and, in some cases, frontotemporal dementia
- Emotional and behavioural change including the following:
  - Emotional lability
  - Significant personality change
  - Disinhibition and impulsivity
  - Perseveration
  - Change in eating behaviour (sweet food preference)
  - Loss of emotional understanding (appear egocentric/selfish)
  - Withdrawn (apathy/failure to initiate)
  - Stereotyped/ritualistic behaviour
  - Behaviour change (MND Association, 2012)

1.5.5 Diagnosing MND

No specific diagnostic tests currently exist, but neurological investigations should normally include EMG, nerve conduction studies, blood tests and investigations that sometimes include MRI/CT scanning, lumbar puncture and muscle biopsy to exclude possibility of other neurological conditions. According to the MND Association (2013), MND can be extremely difficult to diagnose for several reasons:

- It is a comparatively rare disease.
- The early symptoms can be quite slight, such as clumsiness, mild weakness or slightly slurred speech, all of which may have been attributed to a variety of other causes.
- It can be some time before someone feels it necessary to see a GP.
- The disease affects each individual in different ways, not all symptoms may be experienced or appear in the same sequence.

Case study

Evie is 54 years old and lives with her husband Colin. They have three daughters and a son, three of whom live locally within the small village in which Evie grew up. Evie worked in the local school dinner hall and had recently become aware of some loss of function in her left hand. When she examined this a bit more closely, there was a noticeable loss of muscle bulk in her forearm which concerned her. Although seemingly unrelated at the time Evie was aware that at times she seemed to have difficulty forming words and her speech sounded slurred. One evening while Evie was sitting watching television, her husband drew her attention to the muscles in her forearm which were 'flickering' uncontrollably. Evie was aware of this but did not know why this was happening. While Evie did not connect any of the observations, she nevertheless made an appointment with her GP to allay her concerns.

When Evie attended the appointment with her GP, they discussed a number of factors. Evie then recognised that she had been experiencing muscle cramps in her legs but thought this was just due to her exercise regime. Evie remembered that she had tripped on a few occasions recently as her foot seemed to be tired, but this seemed to depend on which shoes she was wearing. Evie had never thought about her swallowing before, but when asked by her GP she realised that her family had made comments about her not taking time to digest her food properly. While at this stage none of this seemed to connect for Evie, there was sufficient evidence for a referral to the neurologist.

Evie attended the neurology appointment with her husband and eldest daughter. Following a thorough clinical examination and history Evie was referred for nerve conduction studies, blood tests, an EMG and an MRI scan. Evie was keen to understand what the neurologist was considering but he was giving very little away at this stage. Evie attended for all her appointments as arranged but in the meantime began to look for information on the Internet regarding the combination of symptoms which were becoming apparent. Evie's aunt had died several years previously from motor neurone disease and Evie was beginning to wonder if there was any connection.

When Evie returned to the neurology clinic, she was given the diagnosis of motor neurone disease. Evie's family were devastated as they had never anticipated this. Evie, being slightly more prepared for this possibility seemed more able to take on board the information which was being shared at this point. Evie was immediately referred to the MND Regional Care Officer and to the multi-disciplinary team. Evie had never heard of occupational therapy but was happy to meet the occupational therapist at the clinic.

When Evie met the occupational therapist she was walking, talking and managing most of the activities within her everyday routine. Her mood was particularly positive and her outlook pragmatic. Evie was aware that her family would require support through this inevitable journey and recognised that her own attitude towards the disease would be pivotal in influencing how they coped with this. Evie shared her concerns about each family member with the occupational therapist and the type of support they would require. Evie also wanted to make her own wishes very clear at this stage while she could.

Evie's difficulties at the time of the occupational therapy referral included loss of power and muscle wastage in her non-dominant hand, fatigue, slow and slurred speech, difficulty with swallowing and shortness of breath. Evie lived in a privately owned home with all facilities upstairs. Evie was no longer working and was visited daily by her family and friends. On one occasion, Evie had 14 visitors coming through her home in one day. While this was really positive in the early stages, this became exhausting for Evie as she became less able. Despite the fairly rapid progression and loss of speech Evie communicated with a communication aid, thanking the occupational therapist on every occasion for her help. Evie developed a relationship with the occupational therapist based on trust and collaboration, which allowed her to share her concerns and frustrations but also her hopes and wishes. Evie communicated with the occupational therapist by text messaging outwith appointments, offering some tremendous insights into her thoughts and feelings given the opportunity to be open and honest in her communications.

Evie continued to deteriorate but remained the matriarch of her family. She experienced some initial difficulties with low mood which required intervention. Her upper limb became weaker, her mobility deteriorated, she continued to experience swallowing difficulties and she lost weight. Her respiratory function deteriorated and she required assistance with breathing at night. Evie's environment was adapted to make life easier for her and her family. They coped with the ongoing deterioration ensuring at all times that Evie's dignity and self-respect were at the forefront of decisions. Evie's concerns throughout her illness were always that of her family and how they would cope after her death. Evie made a lasting impression on everyone she came into contact with, a legacy that her family were proud to hold on to.

1.6 Multiple sclerosis

MS is the most common disabling neurological condition in young adults, affecting around 100 000 people in the United Kingdom. It is most often diagnosed in people between 20 and 40 years of age and affects three times more females than males (MS Society, 2011).

The clinical course of MS may follow a variable pattern over time (Lublin and Reingold, 1996) and is usually characterised by episodic acute periods of worsening, described as attacks, exacerbations or relapse. Typically attacks arise subacutely over hours to days, then plateau and remit partially or fully over the course of weeks or months, either spontaneously or with intervention (Keegan and Noseworthy, 2002). MS is classified according to disease course with each presenting different clinical and epidemiological patterns. The most common classifications of MS include **relapsing-remitting (RRMS)**, **primary progressive (PPMS)**, **secondary progressive (SPMS)** and **benign** MS.

In the early stages following diagnosis people with MS typically present with a relapsing-remitting course in which clearly defined relapses are followed by full or partial recovery. Periods between disease relapses demonstrate a lack of disease progression. After an average of 15 years, the disease develops into a secondary progressive phase during which the course becomes either continuously progressive or progresses with occasional relapses, minor relapses and plateaus. PPMS is characterised by disease progression from onset with occasional plateaus and temporary minor improvements apparent (Lublin and Reingold, 1996).

1.6.1 Body functions

The function of the brain is to interpret sensations and initiate movements and other responses to those sensations. This activity depends upon a highly complex communication system of nerves running from the brain throughout the body via the spinal cord.

1.6.2 Body structures

Each nerve of this complex communication system can be compared to an electric cable. The inner part of the nerve, the axon, is made of conductive tissue and carries messages, or impulses, throughout the body. The axon is surrounded by a layer of fatty substance, the myelin sheath, which protects and insulates the nerve to prevent interference to the impulses passing along it.

Although the aetiology remains unknown, MS is thought to be an autoimmune disorder in which the immune system attacks the myelin sheath around the axons of the central nervous system, which results in plaques or lesions. Damage to the myelin interrupts and disturbs the transfer of information along the axon, with a subsequent failure to carry clear messages to various parts of the body. Axonal damage occurs in addition to demyelination and may be the cause of later permanent disability (Keegan and Noseworthy, 2002; MS Trust website, 2015) as shown in Figure 1.3.

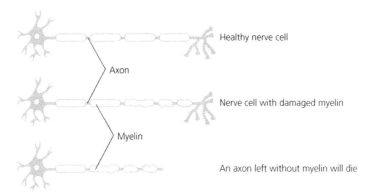

Figure 1.3 Healthy nerve cell and demyelination in MS. (Source: MS Trust website. Reproduced with permission of MS Trust.)

1.6.3 Impairments

There are a number of symptoms or impairments associated with MS, none of which are unique to MS. There is no typical pattern of symptoms that applies to everyone and symptoms can vary in duration and intensity. It is unlikely that a person with MS will develop all of the symptoms listed below (MS Society, 2011):

- Bladder dysfunction
  - Urinary urgency
  - Urinary frequency
- Bowel dysfunction
  - Loss of sensation and neurological control
  - Faecal incontinence
  - Constipation
- Sexual dysfunction
  - Impotence
  - Decreased libido
  - Decreased sensation in the genital area
  - Decreased ability to maintain an erection
  - Absence of ejaculation
  - Decreased lubrication in the vaginal area (MS Trust, 2011)
- Visual disturbances
  - Optic neuritis
  - Diplopia (double vision)
  - Nystagmus
- Fatigue
  - Fatigability: a form of tiredness which occurs after prolonged activity and from which the person recovers after rest
  - Lassitude or a persistent feeling of exhaustion which is not related to rest and sleep
- Pain
  - Neuropathic or neurogenic pain, which is typically described as 'burning, shooting, tingling, stabbing and/or hypersensitivity' (MS Trust, 2011)
  - Nociceptive pain or joint pain
- Spasticity
  - Increased muscle tone due to muscle stretching, peripheral stimulation or infection
  - Involuntary muscle spasms
- Cognitive dysfunction
  - Memory
  - Attention
  - Processing speed
  - Visuospatial abilities
  - Executive functions including planning, problem solving, behavioural regulation, lack of insight, apathy and lack of motivation

- Tremor
  - Postural tremor
  - Kinetic tremor
  - Intention tremor
- Muscle weakness
  - Pattern of weakness usually more distal than proximal
  - Generally greater weakness apparent in the upper limb extensor muscles and the lower limb flexors
  - Footdrop impacting on mobility
- Balance
  - Disturbance of the visual system due to double vision
  - Impaired vestibular processing
  - Damage to the cerebellum resulting in ineffective proprioceptive output
- Vertigo
  - Transient experience or 'feeling of dizziness where the world appears to be spinning' (MS Society, 2013)
  - Inner ear involvement due to nerve damage in the cerebellum or brainstem (MS Society, 2013)
- Altered sensation:
  - Numbness (people often say they feel like they've had a local anaesthetic)
  - Tingling or 'electric shocks'
  - Feeling extremities swollen/ feeling of 'largeness'
  - 'Band-like' sensation around chest or limb
  - 'Burning'
  - Pins and needles
  - Feelings like ants crawling under the skin
  - Lack of awareness of temperature, both hot and cold
  - Transient facial numbness (MS Society, 2011)
- Depression
  - Low mood for more than 2 weeks
  - Variation in mood throughout the day
  - Negative thoughts about self
  - Irrational or illogical thoughts
  - Suicidal ideation
  - Unable to experience pleasure and enjoyment (MS Trust, 2011)
- Emotional and behavioural changes
  - Altered mood in both directions, including euphoria
  - Mood swings
  - Uncontrollable (and often inappropriate) laughing or crying
  - Lack of insight
  - Disinhibition
  - Lack of initiative
  - Withdrawal from usual activities (MS Society, 2011)

- Communication and swallowing
  - Dysarthria or difficulty with speech production and intelligibility
  - Dysphagia or difficulty in swallowing

1.6.4 Diagnosing MS

There is currently no single test or clinical feature which is exclusive to MS, and therefore other conditions must first be eliminated (MS Trust, 2011). The National Institute for Health and Care Excellence (NICE) guideline on the management of MS (NICE, 2014) requires that:

- Only a consultant neurologist should make the diagnosis of MS on the basis of established up-to-date criteria, such as the revised 2010 McDonald criteria (Polman et al., 2011) after:
  - assessing that episodes are consistent with an inflammatory process
  - excluding alternative diagnoses
  - establishing that lesions have developed at different times and are in different anatomical locations for a diagnosis of relapsing-remitting MS
  - establishing progressive neurological deterioration over 1 year or more for a diagnosis of primary progressive MS.

Case study

Brian is 42 years old and was diagnosed with relapsing-remitting multiple sclerosis 8 years ago. Brian went to his GP initially when he had several episodes of double vision, some 'strange' sensations in his right arm and because he was aware that his foot was dragging when he was walking. Brian ran his own business and worked long hours to make this successful. Brian was reluctant to visit his GP as he thought he was just tired from working excessive hours and that his wife was being over dramatic with her concerns.

Brian visited his GP who referred him for a lumbar puncture and an MRI scan. Brian felt this was very thorough, but somewhat unnecessary as he was still determined that his difficulties were due to over exertion at work. Brian attended for the investigations before being invited to attend a follow-up appointment to which he was invited to bring his wife along. Typically, Brian was running late for his appointment, trying to fit in that last minute work appointment.

During this appointment the neurologist advised Brian that there was evidence of plaques forming on his brain which were indicative of multiple sclerosis. He advised Brian that it was not possible to predict how this would progress but that he was presenting with a relapsing-remitting form of MS. Brian was not offered any additional support at this stage and was advised that he could continue to work and drive for the time being. Brian was to arrange a follow up appointment with his GP and the MS specialist nurse.

Brian was naturally devastated at the outcome. However he did not fully understand the diagnosis and did not learn much more from his follow up appointment with his GP. Brian did not alter his lifestyle at all in response to this and continued to work long hours. Brian's wife was particularly concerned about him as she was aware that the happy-go-lucky man she married had become more irritable, always tired, reluctant to go out with friends, and all discussions about starting a family had ceased.

Within 2 months of the diagnosis Brian began to experience increasing difficulties with his walking, numbness in his right arm, and increasing difficulties reading documents at work. Brian felt even more tired than normal. Brian's GP discussed the possibility of disease modifying therapies (DMTs), but Brian said that he did not feel that his symptoms were severe enough at this stage to start on this regime. Brian did not understand the purpose of DMTs and, therefore, was not able to make a fully informed decision about his ongoing care.

An appointment was arranged for Brian with the MS specialist nurse who was able to properly explain the purpose of DMTs once it was established that Brian was a suitable candidate for this intervention. The MS specialist nurse identified some mild cognitive deficits and was aware that Brian was having difficulty with some aspects of his work. Brian was referred to an occupational therapist at this stage.

By the time Brian attended the occupational therapy appointment he had made some fairly significant life decisions. He had decided to sell his business, had put his house on the market and both he and his wife had decided that they would not start a family. Brian was still driving and had not notified DVLA of his diagnosis. Brian presented with difficulties with impaired sensation, reduced mobility, diplopia, urinary urgency, fatigue, mild memory problems and difficulties with executive function. Brian feared for the future as he felt that everything that was important in his life had been slowly eroded and he found it hard to see where his future would lie.

Brian had never heard of occupational therapy before and had no idea why he had been referred. Initially he did not think that occupational therapy would be of any benefit to him until the occupational therapist helped Brian to truly understand what was going on in his life and why this was happening. Together they developed a programme of interventions which helped Brian to continue to engage in meaningful occupations and participate within his wider communities.

1.7 Parkinson's

Parkinson's is predominantly a progressive movement disorder affecting 1 in 500 people. The common age of presentation of symptoms is 65 years; however, Parkinson's can occur in younger people as 20% of those newly diagnosed are under the age of 40 years. Statistically, men are slightly more likely to develop the condition than women (Parkinson's Disease Society, 2007).

1.7.1 Body functions
Dopamine is a major neurotransmitter (a chemical messenger) produced in the basal ganglia which activates receptors in the motor cortex to produce co-ordinated, voluntary and semi-automatic motor skills and movement sequences (Parkinson's Disease Society, 2007). Depletion or deficiency in dopamine can lead to delayed and uncoordinated movements (Parkinson's Disease Society, 2007).

1.7.2 Body structures
Parkinson's is characterised by slow or impoverished movements which impact on the ability to function normally within daily routines. In addition to the

disruption of smooth co-ordinated movement patterns dopamine depletion can also contribute to changes in speed of processing, problem solving, decision-making, visual perception, attention, mood and motivation (Parkinson's Disease Society, 2007). While the cause of Parkinson's remains uncertain like many long-term neurological conditions, environmental factors and genetic suscepti-bility are contributory factors. Approximately 5% of cases of Parkinson's are directly inherited and are usually manifest as early-onset Parkinson's (less than 40 years of age). To date, 10 genes associated with inherited Parkinson's have been identified (Parkinson's Disease Society, 2007).

1.7.3 Impairments

- Bradykinesia or slowness of movement
- Rigidity
- Balance
- Hypokinesia
  - Loss of facial expression
  - Loss of arm swing
- Tremor
  - Apparent at rest
  - Postural tremor
  - Intention tremor
  - Fine rhythmic movement of the thumb and index finger (pill-rolling)
- Freezing
  - Loss of initiation of movement
  - Leads to unpredictable 'on' and 'off' phases
- Pain
  - Neuropathic or 'nerve' pain
  - Nociceptive or musculoskeletal pain
- Restless legs syndrome (RLS)
  - Unpleasant sensations in the legs
  - Uncontrollable urge to move the legs
  - Involuntary jerking of the arms and legs
- Sleep problems
  - Excessive daytime sleepiness
  - Poor sleep regulation
  - Sudden onset of sleep
- Fatigue
  - Fatigability
  - Lassitude
- Bladder problems
  - Nocturia (night-time voids)
  - Urinary urgency
  - Urinary frequency

- Bowel problems
  - Constipation
  - Problems emptying the bowel due to weak abdominal straining and the anal sphincter not relaxing
- Visual problems
  - Difficulty moving eyes
  - Blurred vision
  - Diplopia
  - Dry eyes
  - Involuntary opening and closing of eyelids
- Speech and communication
  - Dysarthria
  - Breathy, nasal or harsh voice
  - Monotony with reduced loudness and pitch range
  - Difficulties with speech initiation
  - Variable rate of delivery of speech
  - Stuttering speech patterns with frequent pauses
  - Short rushes of speech
  - Imprecise consonants
  - Difficulty writing
  - Problems with auditory comprehension
  - Limited eye contact
  - Lack of facial expression (Parkinson's Disease Society, 2007)
- Swallowing
  - Dysphagia
  - Saliva overproduction leading to drooling
  - Weight loss
  - Fear of swallowing
  - A 'gurgly' voice
  - Coughing before, during or after swallowing
  - Difficulty swallowing medications
  - Reduced social contact
  - Recurring chest infections
  - Bronchopneumonia (Parkinson's Disease Society, 2007)
- Cognitive impairment
  - Executive function
  - Planning
  - Sequencing
  - Working memory
- Dementia
  - Parkinson's with dementia (PDD) resulting in the following:
    - Marked cognitive slowing
    - Impairment of visuospatial abilities
    - Memory problems

- Dementia with Lewy bodies (DLB) characterised by the following:
  - Cognitive fluctuations (resembling a chronic confusional state)
  - Visual hallucinations
  - Mild Parkinsonism (Parkinson's Disease Society, 2007)
- Emotional and behavioural change
  - Anxiety
  - Depression
  - Hallucinations

1.7.4 Diagnosing parkinson's

There is no definitive diagnostic test for Parkinson's. Single-photon emission computed topography (SPECT) scanning should be considered for people with tremor where essential tremor cannot be clinically differentiated from Parkinsonism (NICE, 2006).

Case study

James is 58 years old and lives alone, following the death of his mother 4 years previously. James had never married and lived within the family home with his parents all his life. James is a quantity surveyor and worked all over the country depending on where his company placed him. James was a hardworking and loyal employee having worked with the same company for over 30 years. James has many friends and enjoys a very active life including swimming, cycling and running.

Two years ago James became aware of stiffness in his dominant arm. At times there would be a shakiness apparent, but James wasn't aware of this happening at particular times or when doing specific tasks, other than that he was more aware of it when he was relaxing watching the television. James maintained a fairly regular routine, going to bed quite early in the evening so that he could get up early in the morning to exercise before he went into work at least an hour before his starting time. Gradually James felt that he wasn't sleeping as well describing jerkiness in his legs during the night. This woke James up on occasions, but he seemed to settle again once he moved his legs.

During a routine medical assessment at work, James shared his concerns about the stiffness in his arm. James was advised to attend his GP who referred him to a Neurologist. Initially James was advised that he had an essential tremor. James however did not feel reassured by this diagnosis as this did not explain the stiffness in his arm. During a follow-up appointment with the neurologist, however, James was diagnosed with Parkinson's. In addition to the stiffness becoming more apparent in James' upper limb, he had become aware of changes in his posture, his walking was slower and stiffer, he was constipated, had dry eyes and was experiencing difficulties with writing and occasionally choking on his food.

James was referred to a Parkinson's specialist and the multi-disciplinary team, including occupational therapy. The occupational therapist carried out a full assessment of James both in the clinic and within his own home. On assessment it became apparent that James was experiencing a range of difficulties including: standing from a low armchair; preparing and eating food; accessing his shower; loss of confidence in his driving ability; reduced stamina and tolerance in walking. James was climbing into bed on his 'all fours' but could not turn to get into a lying position once he was on the bed. He was lying awake at night worrying that he would need to get up to the toilet as he had difficulty getting back out of bed.

In addition to the practical difficulties James was also experiencing a general loss of confidence reflected in his withdrawal from social activities. He was now on long-term sickness leave from work and was negotiating a medical retirement package with his employer. James was no longer exercising as he found he was particularly stiff in the morning and needed some time before his medication kicked in, allowing him to move more freely. James had notified DVLA of his diagnosis but was no longer driving as his friends had indicated that they felt his driving was unsafe due to his slow decision-making and commented that he was leaving extra distance between other vehicles when he was driving. James felt he did not need to drive and was able to access sufficient support from family and friends when he needed to go anywhere.

James had commenced a medication regime but was experiencing fluctuating levels of ability in response to this. He described episodes of freezing, particularly when going through doorways. This made James feel anxious about his ability to cope, which at times made him feel quite sad. James worried about disease progression as he was a very private man and worried about having to accept support in the form of professional carers coming into his home. James had privately purchased a chair which had been expensive and which was not making it any easier for him to stand up. James was experiencing some difficulties negotiating with his employers due to their apparent lack of understanding about his reasons for being unfit for work.

1.8 Self-evaluation questions

1 What is the economic impact of long-term neurological conditions on health and social care systems?
2 What are the three levels of human functioning within the ICF framework?
3 What are the most common cognitive impairments in HD?
4 What are the most common classifications of MS?
5 What are the key differences between tremor associated with MS and a Parkinsonian tremor?
6 Which of the four neurological conditions – HD, MND, MS and PD – have a genetic inheritance?
7 What is the difference between fatigability and lassitude?
8 What are the main forms of MND?
9 What is the function of dopamine?
10 What are the main causes of depression for people with long-term neurological conditions?

References

Association of British Neurologists (2003) UK neurology – the next 10 years: putting the patient first. London: Association of British Neurologists.

Department of Health (2005) The National Service Framework (NSF) for long term neurological conditions. London: Department of Health.

Huntington's Disease Association (2012) A guide to Huntington's disease for General Practitioners and the Primary Health Care Team. Liverpool: Huntington's Disease Association.

Keegan BM and Noseworthy JH (2002) Multiple sclerosis. Annual Review of Medicine, 53:285–302.

Lublin FD and Reingold SC (1996) Defining the clinical course of multiple sclerosis: results of an international survey. National Multiple Sclerosis Society (USA) Advisory Committee on Clinical Trials of New Agents in Multiple Sclerosis. Neurology, 46(4):907–911.

Motor Neurone Disease (MND) Association (2012) Motor neurone disease: a problem solving approach for General Practitioners and the Primary Health Care Team. Northampton: MND Association.

Motor Neurone Disease (MND) Association (2013) Living with motor neurone disease. Northampton: MND Association.

Multiple Sclerosis (MS) Society (2011) Multiple sclerosis – the quick guide for hospitals, residential homes and nursing homes. London: MS Society.

Multiple Sclerosis (MS) Society (2013) Balance and MS. London: MS Society.

Multiple Sclerosis Trust (2011) Multiple sclerosis information for health and social care professionals, 4th Edition. Hertfordshire: Multiple Sclerosis Trust.

Multiple Sclerosis Trust (2015) Understanding MS: Nerve damage caused by MS. Hertfordshire: Multiple Sclerosis Trust.

Nance M, Paulsen JS, Rosenblatt A and Wheelock V (2013) A physicians guide to the management of Huntington disease, 3rd Edition. Kitchener, ON: Huntington Society of Canada.

National Institute for Health and Care Excellence (NICE) (2006) NICE clinical guideline 35 Parkinson's disease: diagnosis and management in primary and secondary care. London: NICE.

National Institute for Health and Care Excellence (NICE) (2014) NICE clinical guideline 186 MS management: management of MS in primary and secondary care. London: NICE.

Parkinson's Disease Society (2007) The professionals guide to Parkinson's disease. London: Parkinson's Disease Society.

Polman CH, Reingold SC, Banwell B, Clanet M, Cohen JA, Filippi M, Fujihara K, Havrdova E, Hutchinson M, Kappos L, Lublin FD, Montalban X, O'Connor P, Sandberg-Wollheim M, Thompson AJ, Waubant E, Weinshenker B and Wolinsky JS (2011) Diagnostic criteria for multiple sclerosis: 2010 revisions to the McDonald criteria. Annals of Neurology, 69:292–302.

Quarrell O (2008) The facts: Huntington's disease, 2nd Edition. Oxford University Press, Oxford.

World Federation of Occupational Therapists (2011) Statement on occupational therapy. Forrestfield, WA: World Federation of Occupational Therapists.

World Health Organisation (WHO) (2002) Towards a common language for functioning, disability and health: ICF. Geneva: World Health Organisation.

CHAPTER 2

Delivering good quality, safe and effective care

2.1 Introduction

Within the current political and economic climate occupational therapists are increasingly required to work within limited resources and make decisions regarding the most effective interventions to offer people with long-term neurological conditions. This chapter explores the factors that contribute to clinical decision-making and how occupational therapists combine their knowledge of the evidence base, the preferences of people with long-term neurological conditions and an awareness of their own capabilities, in delivering good quality, safe and effective care.

2.2 The strategic context

Strategy or policy offers a political vision which determines the key drivers for change in health and social care. Current policy relating to people with long-term neurological conditions requires the following:
- Delivery of safe and effective programmes of intervention
- Person-centred approaches to care
- Maximising scarce occupational therapy resources to ensure equity of access
- Involvement of people with long-term neurological conditions in the development and design of co-ordinated and integrated occupational therapy services
- Preventative measures to reduce demand and lessen inequalities.

Occupational therapists are required to draw on a range of evidence, guidelines and professional standards to inform their practice and to support their ongoing continuing professional development. The evidence relevant to supporting people with long-term neurological conditions will be presented in a hierarchical structure in this chapter for ease of explanation and clarity although it is recognised that they will be applied within a more integrated approach in practice.

Occupational Therapy and Neurological Conditions, First Edition. Edited by Jenny Preston and Judi Edmans.
© 2016 John Wiley & Sons, Ltd. Published 2016 by John Wiley & Sons, Ltd.

2.2.1 National Service Framework for long-term conditions

The National Service Framework (NSF) is a 10-year strategy to transform the way care services support people with long-term neurological conditions to live as independently as possible (Department of Health, 2005). It sets quality standards for supporting people with long-term conditions. The NSF for long-term conditions was developed to:

- Ensure quick access to specialist neurological expertise for help as close to home as possible
- Support people to live with long term neurological conditions
- Improve their quality of life by providing services to support independent living.

At the heart of the NSF are 11 quality requirements based on currently available evidence, including what people with long-term neurological conditions said about their experiences and needs as follows:

Quality requirement 1: A person-centred service

People with long-term neurological conditions are offered integrated assessment and planning of their health and social care needs. They are to have the information they need to make informed decisions about their care and treatment and, where appropriate, to support them to manage their condition themselves.

Quality requirement 2: Early recognition, prompt diagnosis and treatment

People suspected of having a neurological condition are to have prompt access to specialist neurological expertise for an accurate diagnosis and treatment as close to home as possible.

Quality requirement 3: Emergency and acute management

People needing hospital admission for a neurosurgical or neurological emergency are to be assessed and treated in a timely manner by teams with the appropriate neurological and resuscitation skills and facilities.

Quality requirement 4: Early and specialist rehabilitation

People with long-term neurological conditions who would benefit from rehabilitation are to receive timely, ongoing and high-quality rehabilitation services in hospital or other specialist settings to meet their continuing and changing needs. When ready, they are to receive the help they need to return home for ongoing community rehabilitation and support.

Quality requirement 5: Community rehabilitation and support

People with long-term neurological conditions living at home are to have ongoing access to a comprehensive range of rehabilitation, advice and support to meet their continuing and changing needs, increase their independence and autonomy and help them to live as they wish.

Quality requirement 6: Vocational rehabilitation

People with long-term neurological conditions are to have access to appropriate vocational assessment, rehabilitation and ongoing support, to enable them to find, regain or remain in work and access other occupational and educational opportunities.

Quality requirement 7: Providing equipment and accommodation

People with long-term neurological conditions are to receive timely, appropriate assistive technology/equipment and adaptations to accommodation to support them to live independently, help them with their care, maintain their health and improve their quality of life.

Quality requirement 8: Providing personal care and support

Health and social care services work together to provide care and support to enable people with long term neurological conditions to achieve maximum choice about living independently at home.

Quality requirement 9: Palliative care

People in the later stages of long-term neurological conditions are to receive a comprehensive range of palliative care services when they need them to control symptoms, offer pain relief and meet their needs for personal, social, psychological and spiritual support, in line with the principles of palliative care.

Quality requirement 10: Supporting family and carers

Carers of people with long-term neurological conditions are to have access to appropriate support and services that recognise their needs both in their role as carer and in their own right.

Quality requirement 11: Caring for people with neurological conditions in hospital or other health and social care settings

People with long-term neurological conditions are to have their specific neurological needs met while receiving treatment or care for other reasons in any health or social care setting.

2.2.2 Clinical standards: Neurological Health Standards

The overall aim of NHS Quality Improvement Scotland was to produce standards that will address the patient journey from the point of referral into the service and will result in an improvement in care for all of those suffering from neurological conditions (NHS Quality Improvement Scotland, 2009). The standards were intended to support rather than duplicate existing quality initiatives. The Neurological Health Standards include four generic standards:
- Standard 1: General neurological health services provision
- Standard 2: Access to neurological health services
- Standard 3: Patient encounters in neurological health services
- Standard 4: Management processes in neurological health services

In addition service-specific standards were developed for motor neurone disease (MND), multiple sclerosis (MS) and Parkinson's services with each including three components of access to specialist disease specific services, diagnosis of specific disease, and ongoing management of specific disease. The future vision for neurological health services in Scotland is that 'every patient in Scotland referred with a disorder of the nervous system experiences a quality of care that gives confidence to patient, referrer and provider'.

This will be achieved by ensuring the individual:

- Is assessed by the right person at the right time
- Has timely access to investigations that promote care
- Is encouraged to participate in decision-making on a partnership basis when desired
- Has easy access to information and services that enhance the long-term management of their condition.

2.3 Evidence-based practice

Evidence-based medicine was originally defined as 'the conscientious and judicious use of current best evidence from clinical care research in the management of individual patients' (Sackett et al., 1996). For occupational therapists, practising in an evidence-based way means integrating the best available evidence with clinical expertise and client values in making decisions about individual client care (Sackett et al., 2000) as illustrated in Figure 2.1.

2.3.1 Why do we need evidence-based practice?
- To provide the most effective care and improve client outcomes
- To ensure people with long-term neurological conditions receive the care that fits their needs
- To minimise risk so that benefits outweigh harm
- To increase consistency in the delivery of care
- To ensure interventions are up to date and relevant
- To ensure scarce resources are used wisely (Hoffman et al., 2010).

2.3.2 Finding the best evidence
There are different forms of evidence which can be used to inform neurological practice. However the main forms of scholarly evidence include the following:

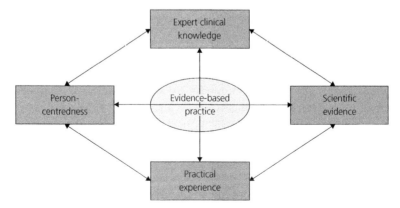

Figure 2.1 Evidence-based practice applied to occupational therapy. (Adapted from Hoffman et al., 2010, Figure 1.1, p. 7. Reproduced with permission of Churchill Livingstone Elsevier.)

- **Books** can vary in quality, so it is important to consider the expertise and reputation of the author; other titles produced by the publisher; the use of references and citations; relevance; and currency to neurological practice (Lou and Durando, 2015).
- **Non-Peer-Reviewed Journals and Professional Magazines** (e.g. OTNews) can be a useful source for current developments and discussions. Generally they are not subject to the same scientific scrutiny as peer-reviewed papers which may impact on the application of the findings to neurological practice. It is not recommended to rely solely on this source of evidence to inform your clinical practice (Lou and Durando, 2015).
- **Peer-Reviewed Journals** (e.g. British Journal of Occupational Therapy) are generally considered more accurate and relevant as they have been subject to a rigorous scrutiny by neurological experts to ensure higher academic quality, including accuracy of content, methodological design and relevance to neurological practice (Lou and Durando, 2015).
- **Clinical guidelines** (e.g. National Institute for Health and Care Excellence (NICE) clinical guidelines) offer a series of systematically developed recommendations on how to care for people with long-term neurological conditions, based on the best available evidence (NICE, 2014). Due to the process of evidence review, however, an absence of occupational therapy evidence in clinical guidelines does not necessarily reflect an absence of effectiveness of interventions (Drummond and Wade, 2014).
- **Practice guidelines** are a set of statements or management strategies developed by expert occupational therapists which outline the most prudent approaches to aspects of neurological practice incorporating evidence where this exists (Bennett and Bennett, 2000).
- **Standards of practice** include statements of principles to enable occupational therapists to monitor and improve their practice and maintain excellence in the quality care for people with long-term neurological conditions. The standards are underpinned by legislation and regulatory and monitoring bodies (College of Occupational Therapists, 2011).

2.3.3 Using electronic databases to find evidence

Electronic databases are collections of published research, scholarly articles, books, dissertations and reports (Lou and Durando, 2015). Access to electronic databases, for example CINAHL, MEDLINE, PsycINFO and the Cochrane Collaboration, requires a username and password which can be obtained through your librarian depending on your institutional subscription. The range of electronic databases has different functions and may identify different resources. Relevant articles can be retrieved through the use of a well-constructed search strategy using subject headings and/or key words. Articles can be reproduced in the form of abstracts or in full-text PDF format. Copyright restrictions apply to both the storage and use of materials which are subsequently downloaded.

2.3.4 Appraising the evidence

The quality of published research varies due to a number of factors such as the design of the study or the standard of the publication. Occupational therapists must evaluate the reliability of evidence before they decide if the results of the study should inform changes to their clinical practice. A range of tools or critical appraisal checklists are available to support the occupational therapist to determine the validity and clinical usefulness of research (Bennett and Bennett, 2000). The most commonly used checklists include those developed by the Critical Appraisal Skills Programme (CASP, 2014) and the McMaster University Centre for Evidence-Based Medicine (CEBM, 2015). The key aims of critical appraisal are to determine the following:

- Are the results of the study valid?
- What are the results?
- How can the results be applied to clinical practice?

Internal Validity refers to the trustworthiness of the results and is determined by the methodological quality of the study (Hoffman et al., 2010). Different criteria apply for determining the validity of different types of study, that is treatment, diagnosis and prognosis (CASP, 2014). Individual studies are ranked within a scale of levels of evidence to determine the strength and quality of the research design and method and whether the outcomes are unlikely to be caused by extraneous variables (Lin et al., 2010). Randomised controlled trials are rated as high internal validity as a result of their design, randomisation and the existence of a control group (Lin et al., 2010). Studies which are considered to be flawed, for example they have not controlled for bias or the results are misleading will not provide high-quality evidence (Bennett and Bennett, 2000; Hoffman et al., 2010).

Clinical Usefulness determines if there is sufficient evidence to integrate the evidence into practice (Lin et al., 2010). Clinical significance relates to the meaningfulness of that change and whether changing practice would bring about substantial benefit to the client.

Applicability determines whether the results of the study can be applied within your practice context, that is can the results be applied to your client population, is it feasible to introduce the intervention within your practice setting and how do the results of the study fit with other available evidence (Coupar and Edmans, 2010).

2.3.5 Implementing findings into clinical practice

Implementation of evidence in clinical practice is a critical part of evidence-based practice and possibly the most challenging component (Lin et al., 2010). It is frequently stated that it takes an average of 17 years for research evidence to reach clinical practice (Morris et al., 2011). Yet changes in the way health and social care is being delivered, for example increasing costs, reduced staffing levels and shorter hospital admissions, require timely incorporation of sufficiently rigorous evidence (Graham et al., 2007; Lin et al., 2010). Even when the best available evidence is known organisational and economic factors can contribute to the challenges occupational therapists face when trying to change established practice (Ilott, 2003).

The key factors which are believed to impact on the incorporation of evidence at the practice level can be defined within three main categories (Lencucha et al., 2007; Upton et al., 2014):

Knowledge and skills
- Limited searching skills
- Limited appraisal skills
- Difficulties understanding research findings
- Poor information technology skills and lack of ability to undertake Web-based literature searches

Resources
- Lack of time to read research and implement findings
- Large caseload, workload pressures and staffing shortages
- Difficulty accessing evidence
- Lack of organisational support

Attitudes
- Perceived lack of evidence to support occupational therapy intervention
- Preference for experience over research evidence
- Reluctance to change practice that has been built up over time
- Tendency to search for evidence that confirms hunches rather than contradict current practice
- Perception that research evidence is difficult to apply to individual clients
- Challenges the competence of individual therapists

2.3.6 Using evidence to inform clinical decisions in occupational therapy

Occupational therapists are required to make complex clinical decisions at all stages of the occupational therapy process (Bennett and Bennett, 2000). This can range from fast, intuitive decisions through to well-reasoned, analytical, evidence-based decisions that drive client care (NHS Education for Scotland, 2015). Occupational therapists apply four strategies when making clinical decisions (Lee and Miller, 2003):
- Decisions made on intuition or based on what feels right or seems reasonable. Such decisions however can be difficult to justify because of their subjective nature despite the fact that they may reflect extensive clinical experience.
- Parsimony is a strategy for choosing between alternative interventions. This strategy is based on an assumption that where two interventions are of potentially equal benefit, then the simpler intervention should be selected.

- Consensual validation reflects the notion that if more than one person concurs with a particular conclusion, then it is more likely to be valid. In clinical practice this often takes the form of peer discussion and consensus of experience.
- Cross-validation seeks to gather a broad range of evidence incorporating multiple decision strategies to reduce bias or subjective interpretation.

Clinical decisions are therefore informed by a range of different types of evidence which reflect the complexity of clinical practice (Lee and Miller, 2003). Evidence-based practice offers a structured approach to clinical decision-making supporting occupational therapists to resolve clinical questions and make informed treatment decisions (Bennett and Bennett, 2000). The process can be summarised through the following five stages (Bannigan, 2007):

1 Formulate a clear clinical question.
2 Find the best evidence.
3 Critically appraise the evidence.
4 Implement useful findings in practice.
5 Evaluate the effectiveness of the new way of working.

2.3.7 Asking clinical questions

Occupational therapists ask clinical questions in relation to many aspects of practice including diagnosis, treatment, prevention, prognosis, client experience and cost-effectiveness (Sackett et al., 1997). Clinicians new to neurological practice are more likely to ask clinical questions that refer to general phenomenon, that is who, what, where, when, how and why, for example 'what is the occupational therapist's role with people with Motor Neurone Disease?' (Lin et al., 2010).

Occupational therapists with greater experience of neurological practice appear more interested in specific questions that relate to interventions and management of neurological conditions (Lin et al., 2010). The most effective way of answering this type of question relies on systematic review or meta-analysis and requires the clinical question to be framed using the PICO format, specifying a **P**opulation or problem, **I**ntervention, **C**omparison intervention (if relevant) and **O**utcome (Lin et al., 2010).

In the context of neurological practice, if the clinical question asks 'Is assessment of a functional task more reliable than the Behavioural Assessment of the Dysexecutive Syndrome (BADS) at identifying executive function impairment in people with Huntington's disease (HD)?' The PICO framework would be applied as follows:

P: clients with HD
I: functional task
C: BADS
O: accurate identification of executive function deficits

A range of examples of clinical questions in relation to neurological practice are included within Table 2.1.

Table 2.1 Examples of neurological clinical questions and recommended levels of evidence.

Question type (generic questions)	Question examples	Hierarchies of evidence (in descending order for each question type)
Diagnostic tests/ assessments: Which is the best diagnostic test/assessment to use and how should it be interpreted? What is the sensitivity and specificity of the test?	What is the accuracy of the Beck Depression Inventory for detecting major depression in HD?	• Systematic review of diagnostic studies • Comparison of diagnostic test and reference standard in a random or consecutive sample • Comparison of diagnostic test and reference standard in non-consecutive sample • Diagnostic study without reference standard • Expert opinion
Treatment: Which treatment is the most effective, and will do more good than harm? When is the optimum time to commence treatment? How long should treatment continue for? What are the possible complications?	For people with Parkinson's, is relaxation therapy in addition to anti-anxiolytics more effective in reducing anxiety compared with medication alone?	• Systematic review of well-designed randomised controlled trials • Well-designed randomised controlled trial (RCT) • Non-randomised trials, single group pre-post, time series, or cohort study • Case-control study • Descriptive studies • Expert opinion
Prevention: How can risk factors for a disease/complication/ occupational status dysfunction be modified?	Does Lycra splinting reduce upper limb tremor in people with MS?	• Same as treatment
Prognosis: What is the client's likely clinical course or consequences of the disease, disability or condition?	What are the strongest predictors of return to work following diagnosis with a progressive neurological condition?	• Systematic review of inception cohort studies • Cohort studies • Case series • Expert opinion
Client's concerns/issues/ feelings: What are the likely issues, concerns, feelings of this client group?	What are the major concerns likely to be for people diagnosed with MND?	• Systematic review • Qualitative or survey study designs from multiple centres or research groups • Expert opinion, including consumers, based on report of expert committees or experience
Economic evaluation: What is the cost-effectiveness, cost benefit, or cost-utility of various treatments?	In clients receiving fatigue management education, is group or individual occupational therapy most cost-effective?	• Systematic review of high quality economic studies • Individual economic study comparing all outcomes against costs • Analysis comparing limited outcomes with cost • Analysis without accurate cost measurement • Expert opinion

Source: Adapted from: Bennett and Bennett, 2000, Table 1, p. 174. Reproduced with permission of John Wiley & Sons.

Table 2.2 Key clinical guidelines for the management of long-term neurological conditions.

Guideline	Recommendations
NICE CG186	**Management of multiple sclerosis in primary and secondary care (NICE, 2014)** This guideline offers best practice advice on the care of adults with multiple sclerosis (MS) including diagnosis, information and support, treatment of relapse and management of MS-related symptoms. The guideline is aimed primarily at services provided within primary and secondary care
NICE CG35	**Parkinson's disease: Diagnosis and management in primary and secondary care (NICE, 2006) (update due 2016)** This guideline offers best practice advice on the care of people with Parkinson's and should be read in conjunction with the national service framework (NSF) for long-term (neurological) conditions (2005)
NICE NG42	**Motor neurone disease: Assessment and management (NICE 2016)** This guideline offers best practice advice on the assessment and management of adults with MND.
SIGN 113	**Diagnosis and pharmacological management of Parkinson's disease: A national clinical guideline (SIGN, 2010)** This guideline provides recommendations based on current evidence for best practice in the diagnosis and pharmacological management of Parkinson's. It includes comparisons of the accuracy of diagnoses carried out by different healthcare professionals as well as the value of different diagnostic tests for differentiating Parkinson's from other associated conditions. It includes a comprehensive assessment of pharmacological management of motor and non-motor symptoms associated with Parkinson's. It also includes a narrative review of qualitative evidence describing the attitudes, beliefs and opinions of clients with Parkinson's

2.4 Clinical guidelines

Clinical guidelines such as those developed by the NICE and the Scottish Intercollegiate Guidelines Network (SIGN) support a consistent approach to care across the multidisciplinary team. They also provide a framework against which practice can be measured (Broughton and Rathbone, 2001). Clinical guidelines can cover any aspect of a condition and may include recommendations about providing information and advice, prevention, diagnosis and longer-term management. Key clinical guidelines relevant to the management of long-term neurological conditions are shown in Table 2.2.

2.5 Practice guidance

Practice guidance documents relevant to long-term neurological conditions include the following:

2.5.1 Occupational therapy in the prevention and management of falls in adults

Written with the collaboration of expert occupational therapists from the College of Occupational Therapists Specialist Section – Older People, this practice guideline aims to support clinical practice and decision-making (College of Occupational Therapists, 2015b). Developed from the best available evidence the guideline provides specific recommendations of the role of occupational therapists within the multi-factorial assessment and intervention required to prevent and manage falls.

2.5.2 Splinting for the prevention and correction of contractures in adults with neurological dysfunction

Written with the collaboration of expert occupational therapists from the College of Occupational Therapists Specialist Section – Neurological Practice and expert physiotherapists on behalf of the Association of Chartered Physiotherapists in Neurology (ACPIN), this practice guideline aims to support clinical practice and decision-making (Kilbride, 2015). Developed from the best available evidence the guideline provides specific recommendations for the use of splinting as an intervention for adults who have, or are at risk of, contractures.

2.5.3 Occupational therapy for people with Parkinson's

Written by expert occupational therapists from the College of Occupational Therapists Specialist Section – Neurological Practice and produced in partnership with Parkinson's UK, these guidelines draw upon relevant knowledge and evidence to describe and inform best practice occupational therapy for people with Parkinson's (Aragon and Kings, 2010). They have been written as an accessible 'pick up and use' guide which includes practical examples of interventions to enable occupational therapists from a diverse variety of health and social care settings to apply new and existing treatments in their day-to-day practice, as well as being of interest to other health professionals, commissioners, service users and carers.

2.5.4 Management of the Ataxias: Towards best clinical practice

Written by Ataxia UK, this document aims to provide recommendations for healthcare professionals on the diagnosis and management of people with ataxia (De Silva et al., 2009). They have been developed through extensive consultation with ataxia specialist neurologists and other healthcare professionals in support with Ataxia UK, the patient support organisation.

2.5.5 Fatigue management for people with multiple sclerosis

Written by the College of Occupational Therapists Specialist Section – Neurological Practice, this publication provides occupational therapists with the theoretical background and evidence base for fatigue management (Harrison, 2007). It includes practical guidance and resources that can be used to implement a fatigue management programme, and it is designed to meet the immediate demand of occupational therapists working with people with MS in both community-based and in-patient rehabilitation settings.

2.5.6 Translating the NICE and NSF guidance into practice: A guide for occupational therapists

This guide for occupational therapists is a result of collaboration between the MS Society and the College of Occupational Therapists (College of Occupational Therapists and MS Society, 2009). Developed by an advisory group of specialist MS occupational therapists, the key aims of the guidance are to:

1 Support occupational therapists in the implementation of the NICE and NSF guidance for the management of MS in primary and secondary care

2 Place the NICE and NSF guidance in the context of everyday occupational therapy practice in MS

3 Pose key questions for occupational therapists in relation to clinical decision-making in MS and provide information for audit purposes

4 Direct occupational therapists to additional information and resources.

2.5.7 Occupational therapy for people with Huntington's disease: Best practice guidelines

These guidelines have been developed as a reference guide for occupational therapists working across Europe in a variety of health, social care and specialty settings (Cook et al., 2012). Many of the recommendations included within this guideline are based on the opinions of highly specialist occupational therapists from within the European Huntington's Disease Network (EHDN) Standards of Care occupational therapists group. The guideline aims to describe and inform contemporary best practice in occupational therapy for people with HD.

2.6 Client expertise in evidence-based practice

Service user experience provides an essential part of the evidence to support health and care interventions (Rose and Gidman, 2010). Just as occupational therapists value their clinical expertise, service users can also contribute their expertise of living with a long-term neurological condition. This combined approach to evidence supports Sackett's et al. (1997) original view that 'evidence based practice requires a bottom-up approach that integrates the best external evidence with individual clinical expertise and service user choice'. Models of partnership and service user engagement will be discussed in more depth in Chapter 3.

2.6.1 Shared decision-making

Regulatory bodies, including the Health and Care Professions Council (HCPC), view shared decision-making as an ethical imperative and expect occupational therapists to work in partnership with their clients, informing and involving them whenever possible (The Kings Fund, 2011). Shared decision-making leads to improved outcomes when compared to more passive models of decision-making (The Kings Fund, 2011).

In shared decision-making the occupational therapist contributes clinical expertise and research evidence to inform treatment options. This is combined with the client's knowledge about the impact of the condition on their daily life, their personal attitude to risk, values and preferences, to reach agreement on the most appropriate care or support strategies (The Kings Fund, 2011). The key principle of a shared decision-making conversation is that it should:

- Support clients to understand and articulate what they want to achieve from the intervention or self-management approach
- Support clients to articulate their current understanding of their condition
- Inform clients about their condition, about the options for intervention or self-management and the benefits of each
- Support clients to understand and articulate their own concept of risk/harm
- Describe what is known about potential risks or harm associated with the intervention
- Ensure that the occupational therapist and the client arrive at a decision based on mutual understanding of this information (The Kings Fund, 2011).

The record of the decision is then formally recorded within the care plan which should be accessible to the client and the occupational therapist and can be used for a number of different purposes:

- As medico-legal record of the shared decision-making process
- To help coordinate care when clients are receiving treatment or support from a range of healthcare professions or agencies
- As a personally held record that can be continually updated to support behaviour change
- To inform a larger-scale commissioning strategy (The Kings Fund, 2011).

2.7 Quality improvement

Quality is defined as 'the degree to which services for individualised populations increase the likelihood of desired health outcomes and are consistent with current professional knowledge' (Institute of Medicine, 1990). Improving quality is about making care:

- **Safe**: avoiding harm to clients from care that is intended to help them
- **Effective**: providing services based on evidence and which produce a clear benefit
- **Person-centred**: establishing a partnership between the client and the occupational therapist to ensure care respects the individuals needs and preferences

- **Timely**: reducing waits and sometimes harmful delays
- **Efficient**: avoiding duplication and waste
- **Equitable**: providing care that does not vary in quality because of personal characteristics.

Quality improvement therefore aims to 'better client experiences and outcomes through changing individual and organisational behaviour using a systematic change method and strategies' (Øvretveit, 2009). There are many improvement models which can be used to improve quality, all of which focus on key aspects of:

- Understanding or defining the problem or aspect of change
- Understanding current models, systems or processes for service delivery
- Choosing the tools to bring about change including leadership, engagement, skills development, occupational therapist and client engagement
- Evaluating and monitoring the impact of a change.

Such an approach is the plan–do–study–act (PDSA) cycles originally developed within industry and now routinely applied to healthcare (Langley et al., 2009), see Figure 2.2.

The PDSA model for improvement is designed to provide a framework for developing, testing and implementing changes that lead to improvement (Centre for Change and Innovation, 2005). The framework includes three key questions and a process for testing change ideas using PDSA cycles:

1 'What are we trying to accomplish?
- Define the problem
- What is causing concern for clients and occupational therapists?

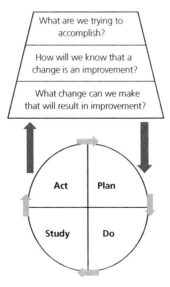

Figure 2.2 Model for improvement. (Source: Langley, 1996, Figure 1.1, p. 24. Reproduced with permission of John Wiley & Sons.)

- What do we already know about this?
- What are we aiming for?

2 How will we know if a change is an improvement?
- What can we measure that will change if the situation is improved?
- How will we obtain this data?
- How accurate are the data?
- What is the best way to display these data?
- Measure the baseline, that is what is happening before the change is implemented?

3 What changes can we make that will result in improvement?
- Changes in clinical practice, for example assessment and interventions
- System and process changes, for example documentation, models of service delivery and the use of resources
- Mechanisms for involving service users in the design and delivery of care.

Plan
- Identify objective
- Identify questions and predictions
- Plan to carry out the cycle (who, where, when).

Do
- Execute the plan
- Document problems and unexpected observations
- Begin data analysis.

Study
- Complete the data analysis
- Compare data to predictions
- Summarise what was learnt.

Act
- What changes are to be made?
- What will the next cycle entail?'

The benefits of this model are (Centre for Change and Innovation, 2005):

- 'It is a simple approach that anyone can apply.
- It reduces risk by starting small.
- It can be used to help plan, develop and implement change.
- It supports cycles of improvement.
- It is highly effective.
- It supports a bottom-up approach to change consistent with systems of continuous improvement.
- It can also be used to facilitate large-scale strategic plans'.

2.8 Health economic evaluation

The aim of an economic evaluation is to determine whether an intervention, programme or treatment is value for money and a good use of scarce resources (Drummond et al., 2001). Economic evaluation is an extremely useful technique especially in the current financial climate where resources are limited and there is less finance available to fund new ideas or service developments.

2.8.1 Key steps of an economic evaluation

'Step 1: Define the question
This involves thinking about the intervention or programme and establishing what you want to show, for example will the intervention improve independence and quality of life?

Step 2: Establish the Population and the Comparators
This step involves determining who the clients are that are affected by the intervention and establish the other options which are available to the client, for example 'do nothing' or 'usual care'.

Step 3: Determine the outcomes
If you want to establish whether your intervention is improving quality of life, you may want to use a quality-of-life questionnaire or scale such as the EQ-5D. If the intervention is about keeping people out of hospital, you may want to think about capturing information around admissions and bed days. Remember with economic evaluation you are always comparing against something, so you also need these outcome measures for the comparator interventions as well.

Step 4: Determine the costs
Unfortunately new ideas or programmes often come with an additional cost, even existing ways of working have a resource cost since when that person is delivering that treatment, they cannot do something else. However it may also be that your intervention is cost saving, so for example a new way of working could allow staff to be used more efficiently. Either way there is a requirement to capture the costs associated with the intervention as well as the comparators and this is a key stage of the evaluation process.

Step 5: Collect the data
Data needs to be captured in a robust way to do justice to your economic evaluation plan.

Step 6: Analysis of results
The information you now have should tell you the cost of the options, so is one option more expensive than the other, and should tell you the outcomes, is one option more effective than the other. If it is the case that your intervention is less costly and produces better outcomes, then that is clearly a cost-effective option

and is said to dominate the alternatives. If the intervention is more costly but produces worse outcome, then that is clearly not cost-effective. If the intervention costs more but produces better outcomes, we have to decide whether the extra cost justifies the additional benefits. In some cases this can be done subjectively by decision-makers, or with certain types of analysis frameworks this can achieved using pre-specified decision-making rules or criteria.

Step 7: Summary of information
This final stage is about reflecting on the results of the evaluation, and you should have a direct answer to the question specified in stage one. If the intervention which prompted the economic evaluation is a good use of resources, then a robust and well planned evaluation will be able to evidence that and support decision-making in the future' (Moseley et al., 2014).

2.9 Professional standards of practice

The College of Occupational Therapists produce a series of professional standards of practice expected of occupational therapists. The standard statements outline a number of criteria against which physical evidence of compliance are sought (College of Occupational Therapists, 2011). The standards include accountability; working in your service users' best interest; consent; the practice and process of occupational therapy; capability, competence and lifelong learning; record keeping; collaborative working; effective communication; and management.

The HCPC (2013), the regulatory body for occupational therapists, sets out standards of proficiency required to determine fitness to practice.

2.10 CPD and lifelong learning

Research, development and evaluation are essential activities which underpin occupational therapy practice. Occupational therapists engage with evidence-based practice primarily at three levels (Eakin et al., 1997):
- As **research consumers** requiring an understanding and ability to critically evaluate research and be able to implement findings
- As **participants in research** requiring participation in research activities including research supervision, presentation at conferences, dissemination through publication, registration on academic programmes with a higher degree component, for example MSc, PhD or Professional Doctorate
- As **proactive researchers** including writing grant applications, accessing funding from grant-awarding bodies, dissemination through publication, strategic and professional research leadership.

Competence in the application of evidence to clinical practice requires that occupational therapists are able to demonstrate the knowledge, skills and behaviours necessary to allow them to fulfil the demands of their role while working within the limits of their professional competence (College of Occupational Therapists, 2011). Continuing professional development (CPD) 'includes a range of learning activities through which occupational therapists maintain and develop throughout their career to ensure that they continue to be able to practise safely, effectively, and legally, within their changing scope of practice' (HCPC, 2013). Learning is recognised as a lifelong process, and all occupational therapists will be required to continue to apply their learning to their practice.

2.10.1 CPD resources

There are a number of resources available which can support occupational therapists to develop the knowledge and skills required to facilitate the delivery of good quality, safe and effective care for people with long-term neurological conditions. These are as follows:

College of Occupational Therapists Resources Supporting Practice – Evidence and Resources (SPEaR) (available at http://www.cot.co.uk/supporting-practice/evidence-and-resources)
- Driving and mobility assessments
- End of life care
- Falls management
- Housing
- MS
- Outcomes
- Parkinson's
- Reablement
- Social care
- Vocational rehabilitation

College of Occupational Therapists briefings (available at http://www.cot.co.uk/briefings/briefings)
- National Service Framework for Long-Term Conditions (College of Occupational Therapists, 2015a)
- Quality and Productivity (College of Occupational Therapists, 2010)
- Assessment and Outcome Measure (College of Occupational Therapists, 2014a)
- Measuring Outcomes (College of Occupational Therapists, 2012b)
- Competencies in Occupational Therapy (College of Occupational Therapists, 2012a)
- Evidence-Based Practice (College of Occupational Therapists, 2014c)
- Including Service Users in Research (College of Occupational Therapists, 2013)
- Research Resources for Occupational Therapists (College of Occupational Therapists, 2014d)
- Applying for Ethics Approval for Research (College of Occupational Therapists, 2014b)

- Motor Neurone Disease: Role of Occupational Therapy (College of Occupational Therapists, 2015c)
- Motor Neurone Disease: Assessment and Outcome Measures (College of Occupational Therapists, 2015d)

Suggested CPD activities
- Attend a research meeting or research seminar.
- Read a research article.
- Contact your library or Research and Development Department to find out what training is available for the development of critical appraisal skills and sign up for a training session.
- Attend or establish a journal club.
- Implement a small test of change using PDSA methodology
- Complete a learning activity from the Effective Practitioner Web-based resource (available at http://www.effectivepractitioner.nes.scot.nhs.uk/learning-and-development/evidence,-research-and-development.aspx).
- Make an appointment with your librarian and find out how they can help you find evidence.
- Volunteer as a participant in a research study or respond to a questionnaire.
- Visit the College of Occupational Therapists website (available at http://www. cot.co.uk/research-development/research-resources).
- Participate in an interactive workshop or a webinar.
- Capture a 'patient story' and consider how you could improve their experience.
- Join the College of Occupational Therapists Specialist Section – Neurological Practice (available at http://www.cot.co.uk/cotss-neurological-practice/become-member).
- Register for a research methods module at your local university.
- Apply to join the Regional Ethics Committee.

2.11 Self-evaluation questions

1 Why is it important to deliver good quality, safe and effective care?
2 What are the current political drivers impacting on the delivery of care to people with long-term neurological conditions?
3 Name three reasons why we need evidence-based practice.
4 What are the four types of clinical decision-making in occupational therapy practice?
5 Name the five stages of evidence-based practice.
6 Where would you find evidence relevant to occupational therapy practice?
7 What are the six dimensions of quality in health and social care?
8 What does PDSA stand for?
9 How can health economics impact on occupational therapy service delivery?
10 Name the three levels of engagement with research as an occupational therapist.

References

Aragon A and Kings J (2010) Occupational therapy for people with Parkinson's: best practice guidelines. London: College of Occupational Therapists and Parkinson's UK.

Bannigan K (2007) Making sense of research utilisation. In Creek J and Lawson-Porter A (Eds) Contemporary issues in occupational therapy: reasoning and reflection. Chichester: John Wiley & Sons, Ltd, pp. 189–216.

Bennett S and Bennett JW (2000) The process of evidence-based practice in occupational therapy: informing clinical decisions. Australian Occupational Therapy Journal, 47(4):171–180.

Broughton R and Rathbone B (2001) What makes a good clinical guideline? Kent: Hayward Medical Communications.

Centre for Change and Innovation (2005) A guide to service improvement. Edinburgh: Scottish Executive.

Centre for Evidence Based Medicine (2015) Critical appraisal resources. Hamilton, ON: McMaster University.

College of Occupational Therapists, Multiple Sclerosis Society (2009) Translating the NICE and NSF guidance into practice: a guide for occupational therapists. London: College of Occupational Therapists.

College of Occupational Therapists (2010) COT/BAOT briefing 128: quality and productivity. London: College of Occupational Therapists.

College of Occupational Therapists (2011) Professional standards for occupational therapy practice. London: College of Occupational Therapists.

College of Occupational Therapists (2012a) Management briefing: competencies in occupational therapy. London: College of Occupational Therapists.

College of Occupational Therapists (2012b) Research briefing: measuring outcomes. London: College of Occupational Therapists.

College of Occupational Therapists (2013) Research briefing: including service users in research. London: College of Occupational Therapists.

College of Occupational Therapists (2014a) Good practice briefing: assessment and outcome measure. London: College of Occupational Therapists.

College of Occupational Therapists (2014b) Research briefing: applying for ethics approval for research. London: College of Occupational Therapists.

College of Occupational Therapists (2014c) Research briefing: evidence based practice. London: College of Occupational Therapists.

College of Occupational Therapists (2014d) Research briefing: research resources for occupational therapists. London: College of Occupational Therapists.

College of Occupational Therapists (2015a) Legislation, policy and strategy briefing: National Service Framework for Long Term Conditions. London: College of Occupational Therapists.

College of Occupational Therapists (2015b) Occupational therapy in the prevention and management of falls in adults. London: College of Occupational Therapists.

College of Occupational Therapists (2015c) Practice briefing: motor neurone disease: role of occupational therapy. London: College of Occupational Therapists.

College of Occupational Therapists (2015d) Practice briefing: motor neurone disease: assessment and outcome measures. London: College of Occupational Therapists.

Cook C, Page K, Wagstaff A, Simpson S and Rae D; on behalf of the contributing members of the European Huntington's Disease Networks Standards of Care Occupational Therapist Group (2012) Development of guidelines for occupational therapy in Huntington's disease. Future Medicine, 2(1):79–87.

Coupar F and Edmans J (2010) Evaluation. In Edmans J (Ed.) Occupational therapy and stroke, 2nd Edition. Chichester: Wiley-Blackwell, pp. 191–207.

Critical Appraisal Skills Programme (CASP) (2014) CASP checklists (URL used) Oxford: CASP UK. Hamilton, ON: McMaster University. Available at http://fhswedge.csu.mcmaster.ca/cepftp/qasite/CriticalAppraisal.html (Accessed 28 October 2015).

Department of Health (2005) The National Service Framework for Long Term Conditions. London: Department of Health.

De Silva R, Giunti P, Greenfield J and Hunt B (2009) Management of the Ataxias: towards best clinical practice. London: Ataxia UK.

Drummond A and Wade D (2014) National Institute for Health and Care Excellence stroke rehabilitation guidance – is it useful, usable and based on best evidence? Clinical Rehabilitation, 28(6):523–529.

Drummond MF, O'Brien B, Stoddart GL and Torrance GW (2001) Methods for the economic evaluation of health care programmes, 2nd Edition. Oxford: Oxford University Press.

Eakin P, Ballinger C, Nicol M, Walker M, Alsop A and Ilott I (1997) College of occupational therapists: research and development strategy. British Journal of Occupational Therapy, 60(11):484–486.

Graham ID, Tetroe J and the Knowledge Translation Theories Research Group (2007) Some theoretical underpinnings of knowledge translation. Academic Emergency Medicine, 14:936–941.

Harrison S (2007) Fatigue management for people with multiple sclerosis, 2nd Edition. London: College of Occupational Therapists.

Health and Care Professions Council (HCPC) (2013) Standards of proficiency. London: Health and Care Professions Council.

Hoffman T, Bennett S and Del Mar C (2010) Introduction to evidence based practice. In Hoffman T, Bennett S and Del Mar C (Eds) Evidence based practice: across the health professions. Sydney: Churchill Livingstone Elsevier, pp. 1–16.

Ilott I (2003) Challenging the rhetoric and reality: only an individual and systematic approach will work for evidence based occupational therapy. The American Journal of Occupational Therapy, 57(3):351–354.

Institute of Medicine (1990) Crossing the quality chasm: a new health system for the 21st century. Washington, DC: National Academy Press, pp. 244.

Kilbride C (2015) Splinting for the prevention and correction of contractures in adults with neurological dysfunction: practice guideline for occupational therapists and physiotherapists. London: College of Occupational Therapists.

Langley GJ (1996) The improvement guide: a practical approach to enhancing organisational performance. San Francisco, CA: Jossey-Bass.

Langley GL, Moen R, Nolan KM, Nolan TW, Norman CL, Provost LP (2009) The improvement guide: a practical approach to enhancing organizational performance, 2nd Edition. San Francisco, CA: Jossey-Bass.

Lee CJ and Miller LT (2003) The process of evidence-based clinical decision making in occupational therapy. The American Journal of Occupational Therapy, 57(4):473–477.

Lencucha R, Kothari A and Rouse MJ (2007) Knowledge translation: a concept for occupational therapy. The American Journal of Occupational Therapy, 61(5):593–596.

Lin SH, Murphy SL and Robinson JC (2010) Facilitating evidence-based practice: process, strategies and resources. The American Journal of Occupational Therapy, 64(1):164–171.

Lou JQ and Durando P (2015) Asking clinical questions and searching for the evidence. In Law M and MacDermid J (Eds) Evidence-based rehabilitation: a guide to practice, 3rd Edition. Thorofare, NJ: Slack Incorporated, pp. 105–128.

Morris Z, Wooding S and Grant J (2011) The answer is 17 years, what is the question: understanding time lags in translational research. Journal of the Royal Society of Medicine, 104:510–520.

Moseley O, McKaig S and Preston J (2014) Economic evaluation – key steps. London: College of Occupational Therapists. Available at http://www.cot.co.uk/areas-practice/cost-effectiveness-and-ot (Accessed 28 October 2015).

NHS Education for Scotland (NES) (2015) Clinical decision making. Edinburgh: NHS Education for Scotland. Available at http://www.effectivepractitioner.nes.scot.nhs.uk/learning-and-development/learning-resources/clinical-decision-making.aspx (Accessed 28 October 2015).

NHS Quality Improvement Scotland (2009) Clinical standards: neurological health services. Edinburgh: NHS Quality Improvement Scotland.

National Institute for Health and Care Excellence (NICE) (2006) NICE CG35, Parkinson's disease: Diagnosis and management in primary and secondary care. London: National Institute for Health and Clinical Excellence.

National Institute for Health and Care Excellence (NICE) (2016) NICE NG42, Motor neurone disease: assessment and management. London: National Institute for Health and Clinical Excellence.

National Institute for Health and Care Excellence (NICE) (2014) NICE CG186, multiple sclerosis: management of multiple sclerosis in primary and secondary care. London: National Institute for Health and Clinical Excellence.

Øvretveit J (2009) Does improving quality save money? A review of the evidence of which improvements to quality reduce costs to health service providers. London: The Health Foundation.

Rose P and Gidman J (2010) Evidence-based practice within values-based care. In McCarthy J and Rose P (Eds) Values-based health and social care: beyond evidence-based practice. London: Sage.

Sackett D, Rosenberg W, Gray J, Haynes R and Richardson W (1996) Evidence based medicine: what it is and what it isn't: it's about integrating individual clinical expertise and the best external evidence. British Medical Journal, 312:71–72.

Sackett DL, Richardson WS, Rosenberg W and Haynes RB (1997) Evidence-based medicine: how to practice and teach EBM. Edinburgh: Churchill Livingstone.

Sackett DL, Strauss SE, Richardson WS, Rosenberg W and Haynes RB (2000) Evidence-based medicine: how to practice and teach EBM, 2nd Edition. London: Churchill Livingstone.

Scottish Intercollegiate Guidelines Network (SIGN) (2010) SIGN 113 diagnosis and pharmaco-logical management of Parkinson's disease: a national clinical guideline. Edinburgh: Scottish Intercollegiate Guidelines Network.

The Kings Fund (2011) Making shared decision making a reality: no decision about me, without me. London: The Kings Fund.

Upton D, Stephens D, Williams B and Scurlock-Evans L (2014) Occupational therapists' attitudes, knowledge, and implementation of evidence-based practice: a systematic review of published research. British Journal of Occupational Therapy, 77(1):24–38.

CHAPTER 3

Person-centredness and long-term neurological conditions

3.1 Introduction

Person-centredness relates to treating people with dignity, compassion and respect and as such aligns to the underlying philosophies of occupational therapy. However, the delivery of care which is developed in partnership with people living with a long-term neurological condition, in response to their individual and constantly changing needs, can be challenging for occupational therapists. In this chapter we explore the key principles along with the barriers to delivering person-centred care and offer some practical guidance for occupational therapists moving towards more collaborative models of care.

3.2 Person-centredness

3.2.1 What is person-centred care?

Person-centred care can be defined as 'a partnership among practitioners, clients and their families to ensure that decisions respect clients' wants, needs and preferences and that clients have the education and support they need to make decisions and participate in their own care' (Institute of Medicine, 2001a). Person-centredness assumes that the person living with a long-term neurological condition has the ability to decide their own needs and expectations and that they are able to make decisions and choices about what they need and want (Lutz and Bowers, 2000). The underlying philosophy of person-centred care is about considering the client's opinions and circumstances in the decision-making process and goes well 'beyond simply setting goals with the client' (Ponte et al., 2003).

The underlying principles of person-centredness include care that is personalised, co-ordinated and enabling while ensuring the person is treated with dignity, compassion and respect (The Health Foundation, 2014). Person-centredness requires the occupational therapist to practise in a style which is responsive to the client's needs and wishes through a process of interaction in

Occupational Therapy and Neurological Conditions, First Edition. Edited by Jenny Preston and Judi Edmans.
© 2016 John Wiley & Sons, Ltd. Published 2016 by John Wiley & Sons, Ltd.

which the client and the occupational therapist are constantly influencing each other (Mead and Bower, 2000). The role of the occupational therapist within a person-centred care model is to demonstrate a willingness to understand the wider aspects of neurological disability, appreciative of the challenges from a holistic perspective (Mead and Bower, 2000). Evidence suggests that as client engagement increases, staff performance and morale see a corresponding increase (Finset, 2011; The Kings Fund, 2012).

Developed within a biopsychosocial framework person-centred care seeks to move beyond the understanding of the client within the more conventional biomedical model (Mead and Bower, 2000).

3.2.2 Medical model of care

The underlying principles of the medical model of care have developed within a scientific process which recognises and describes symptoms leading to an accurate diagnosis and the selection of appropriate therapy to restore or improve the client's problems (Neighbour, 1987). Informed by the best available evidence, occupational therapists practising within a medical model offer the person living with a long-term neurological condition specific expertise and advise to overcome their problems or difficulties.

For occupational therapists practising within a medical model of care there are five key stages to the occupational therapy process:

1 **Problem identification**: this is the starting point of the intervention sequence and is intended to gather information which helps understand the nature of the problem, particularly in relation to normal and abnormal functioning, for example range of movement, tremor and memory.

2 **Problem analysis**: once a problem has been identified, it needs to be understood in relation to the client's current situation. The occupational therapist will attempt to define the problem in relation to the client's overall level of functioning, for example increased tone leading to difficulty getting in and out of bed.

3 **Decision-making**: during this phase decisions will be made regarding the desired outcome, and the occupational therapist will begin to problem solve potential solutions and make decisions on the most appropriate approach to overcome the difficulties, for example provision of equipment or specific interventions, such as fatigue management and splinting.

4 **Treatment implementation**: an action plan is developed and implemented based on the best available evidence. The client will be advised of the expectations and any risks associated with the intervention and the potential outcomes.

5 **Evaluation**: the effectiveness of the intervention is measured against the desired outcome and adjusted accordingly. The success of an intervention may be determined by the level of engagement or compliance by the client.

3.2.3 Social model of disability

The social model of disability provides a structure to help occupational therapists understand how disability can limit opportunities for participation in the wider community (Shaw, 2001). It is underpinned by a belief that disability itself is not a restriction to participation, but it is the barriers imposed by society, which create unnecessary isolation and exclusion (Oliver, 1996). It distinguishes between impairment and disability, that is the relationship between a person with impairment and society (Shakespeare and Watson, 2002).

The social model of disability supports people living with a long-term neurological condition to 'achieve the lifestyle of their choice,' recognising the contribution of the occupational therapist as a resource offering knowledge and expertise (Picking, 2000). It has been influential in the development of policy and strategy promoting a culture of social and societal change including equal opportunities and wider accessibility within the built environment (Shakespeare and Watson, 2002).

3.3 Client-centred practice

The concept of client-centred practice is well established within the theoretical models of occupational therapy. The earliest models, described through the work of the Canadian Association of Occupational Therapists and Department of National Health and Welfare (1983), recognised a need by clients for greater autonomy and control over their health conditions (Law et al., 1995). However as the models of client-centred practice have evolved, the key principles have been adopted within the wider care context to reflect and support people to develop the knowledge, skills and confidence they need to more effectively manage and make informed decisions about their health and well-being (The Health Foundation, 2014).

Client-centred practice remains the predominant language in occupational therapy and has developed from the underlying principles of (Law et al., 1995):

1 **Autonomy and choice**: recognising that every person brings a level of expertise developed from their own experience of living with a long-term neurological condition
2 **Partnership and responsibility**: reflecting the visions and values of the person living with a long-term neurological condition
3 **Enablement**: supporting a shift from a deficit model of care to an approach focussing on strengths and supports within natural communities
4 **Context**: recognising the impact of roles, interests, environments and cultures on occupational performance
5 **Accessibility and flexibility**: developing services around the needs of the person living with a long-term neurological condition
6 **Respect for diversity**: acknowledging the importance for occupational therapists to recognise their own values and not to impose these values on clients.

Client-centred practice is both a conceptual framework and a behavioural approach which impacts on the occupational therapy process, that is the sequence of actions which an occupational therapist undertakes to decide on the most appropriate intervention (Hagedorn, 1997). Traditionally occupational therapists have taken an active role in the assessment and identification of problems before deciding on the most appropriate interventions and the desired outcomes (Hagedorn, 1997; Law et al., 1995). In client-centred practice, the person living with a long-term neurological condition assumes a more active role in defining both the goals and the desired outcomes of intervention (Law et al., 1995). The role of the occupational therapist shifts to one of facilitator in working with the person living with a long-term neurological condition to find the means to achieve those goals (Kaplan, 1991).

Within a client-centred model of care the occupational therapist is required to follow a structured process to fully understand the needs of the person living with a long-term neurological condition. The Canadian Practice Process Framework (CPPF) offers a client-centred approach to the occupational therapy process (Davis et al., 2007; Table 3.1).

Stewart et al. (1995) outlined a model of person-centred care with six key stages which, although not specific to occupational therapy, provides a framework to facilitate a person-centred approach:

1 Exploring both the disease and the illness experience
2 Understanding the whole person
3 Finding common ground regarding management
4 Incorporating illness prevention and health promotion
5 Enhancing the therapist–client relationship
6 Being 'realistic' about personal limitations and issues such as the availability of time and resources.

Each stage of this model will be considered within the context of occupational therapy practice and practical guidance, and resources will be identified to support the occupational therapist to develop the knowledge, skills and behaviours required to successfully deliver person-centred care to people living with a long-term neurological condition.

3.3.1 Exploring both the disease and the illness experience

The process of engaging the client in a conversation about their life requires careful planning and preparation on behalf of the occupational therapist. Key factors which need to be considered include the following:

- **Selecting the most appropriate environment** should ideally be determined through agreement between the client and the occupational therapist. Although there is an increasing shift in the balance of care into the community, the occupational therapist should not assume that the client will wish to be visited within their own home. Preston et al. (2012) identified feelings of intrusion and intimidation when occupational therapists visited clients within their own homes.

Table 3.1 The Canadian Practice Process Framework.

The Canadian Process Practice Framework (CPPF): Eight action points at a glance

Action points	Key enablement skills and actions
Enter/initiate	• Call to action: Advocate for the client and occupational therapy to create positive first point of contact with client based on a referral, contract request, or the occupational therapists' recognition of real or potential occupational challenges with individual, family, group, community, organisation or population clients. • Consult to decide whether to continue or not with practice process. • Educate and collaborate to establish and document consent.
Set the stage	• Engage client to clarify values, beliefs, assumptions, expectations, desires. • Collaborate to mediate/negotiate common ground or agree not to continue. • Adapt ground rules to the situation, build rapport, foster client readiness to proceed. • Explicate mutual expectations and document the 'stage' set. • Collaborate to identify priority occupational issues (OIs) and possible occupational goals (OGs)
Assess/evaluate	With client participation and power-sharing as much as possible or desired: • Assess (sometimes called 'evaluate') occupational status, dreams and potential for change. • Consult with the client and others, use specialized skills to assess/evaluate and analyse spirituality, person and environmental influences on occupations. • Coordinate analysis of data and consider all perspectives to interpret findings. • Formulate and document possible recommendations based on best explanations.
Agree on objectives and plan	With client participation and power-sharing as much as possible or desired: • Collaborate to identify priority occupational issues for the agreement in light of assessment/evaluation. • Design/build plan, negotiate agreement on occupational goal, objectives, and plan within time, space and resource boundaries, and within contexts using requisite elements.
Implement the plan	With client participation and power-sharing as much as possible or desired: • Engage client through occupation to implement and document process. • Specialize in program frame of reference as appropriate to effect of prevent change.
Monitor and modify	With client participation and power-sharing as much as possible or desired: • Consult, collaborate, advocate, educate and engage client and others to enable success. • Adapt or redesign plan as needed in monitoring progress through formative evaluation.
Evaluate outcome	With client participation and power-sharing as much as possible or desired: • Re-assess/evaluate occupational challenges and compare with initial findings. • Document and disseminate findings and recommendations for next steps.
Conclude/exit	With client participation and power-sharing as much as possible or desired: • Communicate conclusion of interaction between client and therapist. • Document conclusion/exit and disseminate information for coordinated transfer or re-entry.

Source: Davis et al. (2007), Table 10.1, p. 251. Reproduced with permission of Canadian Association of Occupational Therapists CAOT Publications ACE.

There was also, on occasions, a sense of feeling disloyal to family and friends when discussions took place within the participants' own homes with some participants preferring to create some distance between their personal spaces and their discussions about living with a long-term neurological condition (Preston et al., 2012).

- **Resource availability** includes the staff resource but should also consider the more practical aspects of travelling for appointments, including distance and journey time in addition to the time of the day. For some people living with a long-term neurological condition, it may take a long time to get prepared in the morning and they will therefore require appointments later in the day. Alternatively, aspects of fatigue may require that the appointment is scheduled earlier in the day. Such variation will be client-determined and needs to be considered within a person-centred approach.

- **Aspects of privacy** need to be taken into consideration as the client needs to feel safe to engage in discussion before disclosure can occur. Discussion regarding the presence of family and friends when exploring occupational needs is fundamental in ensuring client privacy and safety. People living with a long-term neurological condition may seek to protect both themselves and others from the reality of their situation, and the occupational therapist needs to be prepared to experience a range of emotions as the client relives the process of receiving a life-changing diagnosis (Preston et al., 2012).

- **Starting a conversation** should be structured to allow the person living with a long-term neurological condition to share their thoughts and opinions in relation to their occupational needs. The occupational therapist should explore the client's situation initially through the use of open-ended questions. The use of conversation tools, for example 5 'Must Do With Me' elements (Person Centred Health and Care Collaborative, 2014) can be helpful to provide some structure for occupational therapists less comfortable with a more narrative approach to assessment and evaluation. It is important that the occupational therapist engages with the conversation while at the same time maintaining silence to allow clients the time to express themselves (Howie et al., 2004). Particular skills are required to develop an ability to actively listen and 'hear' what is being said. Ideally the conversation should be constructed to allow the client the opportunity to elaborate and discuss the areas that that they choose (Morgan, 2002). Narrative conversations are not about offering advice, solutions or opinions but are intended to provide valuable insights into the daily lives of people living with long-term neurological conditions to accurately determine their occupational needs (Morgan, 2002).

3.3.2 Understanding the whole person

Conceptual models of occupational therapy facilitate an understanding of the person living with a long-term neurological condition within the context of the person–environment–occupation–performance in an attempt to gain insight into the whole person. Specific instruments, such as the Canadian Occupational Performance Measure (COPM) (Law et al., 1990) and Model of Human Occupation Screening Tool (MOHOST) (Parkinson et al., 2006) (see Chapter 6), can be used to support the development of a holistic assessment. A flexible approach to the use of assessment and interventions should be considered which value and respect the client's contribution. Careful use of questions such as 'What matters to you?', 'Who matters to you?' and 'What information do you need?' (Person Centred Health and Care Collaborative, 2014) facilitate conversations that enable clients as interactive partners (Kennedy, 2003). People living with a long-term neurological condition want to be listened to carefully regarding their welfare, wishes, values and interests and wish to be viewed and treated as a person rather than a 'patient with a specific condition' (Bolmsjö, 2001).

3.3.3 Finding common ground regarding management

Integrating evidence-based practice and person-centred care requires the occupational therapist to combine knowledge of the best available interventions with the needs and wishes of the person living with a long-term neurological condition. The processes for identifying the best available evidence are discussed in Chapter 2. Within an integrated approach to care, people living with a long-term neurological condition should contribute to the discussion and participate in the decision-making process regarding the selection and implementation of interventions (Sidani et al., 2006). This can be achieved through the following process:

- **Generation of intervention description**: The occupational therapist should present a clear description of the intervention options. This should include the name of the intervention, the goal to be achieved further to collaborative agreement, the nature of the activities to be performed by the client and the occupational therapist, the dose or method of delivery, the expected outcomes and any potential benefits and risks (Sidani et al., 2006). This information should be presented in terms that are simple to understand and where relevant in an easy-to-read format (Sidani et al., 2006).
- **Eliciting preferences:** The principles of a shared decision-making conversation are that it should support the person living with a long-term neurological condition to articulate their current understanding of their condition, understand and articulate what they want to achieve from the intervention, understand the options and arrive at a decision based on mutual understanding of the information (The Kings Fund, 2011). Understanding the client perspective allows the occupational therapist to give treatment options congruent with the client's needs and values (Robinson et al., 2008).
- **Adherence and compliance:** Client involvement in decision-making is linked to improved adherence to treatment, increased satisfaction with care, achievement of desired outcomes and development of a trusting relationship between the occupational therapist and the person living with a long-term neurological condition (Sidani et al., 2006).

3.3.4 Incorporating illness prevention and health promotion

People living with a long-term neurological condition should be encouraged to be active partners in the management of their disease and to take steps to prevent the development of secondary complications wherever possible.

Health promotion aims to promote health giving behaviours through enabling people living with a long-term neurological condition to 'increase control over, and to improve their health' (World Health Organisation, 1986). Health promotion is primarily aimed at:

- Promoting physical activity
- Smoking cessation
- Reduction in substance misuse including alcohol
- Obesity
- Stress reduction.

Behavioural change is most likely to occur when occupational therapists and people living with a long-term neurological condition work in partnership to remove social, financial and environmental barriers that prevent people from making positive changes about their lives (National Institute for Health and Care Excellence [NICE], 2007).

3.3.5 Enhancing the therapist-client relationship

A working alliance is developed and maintained through active negotiation at the start of the interaction between the client and the occupational therapist and is continually reviewed and renegotiated thereafter (Polatajko et al., 2015). Considerable effort is therefore required in building a relationship with the client developed from a position of mutual trust and respect and which supports questioning and learning from each other. Within a person-centred model of care both the occupational therapist and the person living with a long-term neurological condition are experts in their own fields, the occupational therapist in matters of occupation and the person living with the long-term neurological condition in the experience of feelings, fears, hopes and desires (Kennedy, 2003).

Skills required for delivering client-centred practice include the following:

- **Authenticity**: This is an ability to practice within a desired set of standards or criteria for self-judgement demonstrating a commitment to reconcile the occupational therapists' own values with the values of the profession (Polatajko et al., 2015).
- **Empathy:** This includes humaneness, for example warmth and respect (Mead and Bower, 2000). The empathic occupational therapist will listen for and adjust to personal meanings using techniques of rephrasing to check understanding with the person living with a long-term neurological condition (Polatajko et al., 2015). The use of open-ended questions allows the client to tell their story in their own words.
- **Reflexivity:** This involves an understanding of how one's self as an occupational therapist can greatly influence the outcomes of people living with a long-term neurological condition (Polatajko et al., 2015). The occupational therapist is

required to critically review their own actions and interactions and alter behaviour accordingly (Polatajko et al., 2015). Actions based on broad assumptions about clients can lead to weaker alliances between the occupational therapist and the person living with a long-term neurological condition (Polatajko et al., 2015).

- **Responsible collaboration:** Within a collaborative model of care the occupational therapist should not attempt to make all decisions for therapy as this will not enable the development of a strong working alliance and will diminish occupational engagement outcomes (Polatajko et al., 2015). The occupational therapist should negotiate roles and responsibilities with the client, outline parameters of the relationship, be transparent with all actions, listen to client successes and concerns and encourage client participation in the process (Polatajko et al., 2015).

- **Enablement:** This requires the occupational therapist to facilitate and support people living with a long-term neurological condition to recognise their capacities and strengths; celebrate and reward success; convey positive, compelling and consistent messages pertaining to the client's occupational challenges; and help clients realise their key role in the collaboration (Polatajko et al., 2015).

3.3.6 Being 'realistic' about personal limitations and issues such as the availability of time and resources

A person-centred approach to care supports the development of collaborative plans which are uniquely adapted to each person living with a long-term neurological condition (Malec, 1999). However as resources, and indeed the life expectancy, for some people living with a long-term neurological condition may be limited, they must be supported to make decisions about how to make best use of those resources (Wrosch et al., 2003). There may be occasions when the person living with a long-term neurological condition has been engaged in a meaningful occupation or role and the time comes when this is no longer worth sustaining given the multiple constraints on the person's life, or the changing nature of their underlying condition. In such situations, the activity or goal must be abandoned. This allows the person to apply their resources, perhaps to better effect within other domains of their life (Wrosch et al., 2003).

Aspects of motivation, emotion and personal identity also impact on the attainment of goals (Siegert et al., 2004). People living with a long-term neurological condition are more likely to engage in goal-directed behaviours when the perceived complexity of the task is related to their perception of their own ability. Perceived lack of progress towards goal attainment may lead to goal disengagement (Siegert et al., 2004). Occupational therapists should support people living with a long-term neurological condition to focus on aspirations and future development but crucially to recognise which goals to give up and when (Schulz and Heckhausen, 1996).

Determination of collaborative plans also requires recognition that the person living with a long-term neurological condition may reflect a heightened awareness of difficulties due to the impact of cognitive impairment, fatigue, anxiety and depression (Preston et al., 2013). This heightened awareness may reflect the internal experience and the personal significance of change which leads to a greater awareness of difficulties and limitations. Often slow, insidious progression is not acknowledged in the same way by families and carers as they adapt and adjust accordingly.

Barriers to delivering client-centred practice
- Some people living with a long-term neurological condition may be reluctant to assume responsibility for their care.
- The process of giving power/control to the person living with a long-term neurological condition threatens the traditional view of the therapist as expert and may elicit feelings of discomfort.
- Separating personal and professional values from client values can be challenging.
- Organisational barriers such as the dominance of the medical model.
- Perceptions of lack of time.
- Lack of desire to move to a client-centred model.
- Concerns that client-centred practice is too demanding for some clients and that the person living with a long-term neurological condition will choose unsafe or inappropriate goals.
- Difficulties facilitating the client's goal identification (Law et al., 1995; Sumison and Smyth, 2000).

3.4 Self-management

Several definitions of self-management exist, but in general self-management can be defined as 'the individual's ability to manage the symptoms, treatment, physical and psychosocial consequences and lifestyle changes inherent in living with a chronic condition' (Barlow, 2001). Fundamentally self-management facilitates more active involvement of the person living with a long-term neurological condition by shifting day-to-day responsibility for disease management from the occupational therapist to the individual (Barlow et al., 2002).

Self-management is generally considered within three core domains of disease management, behavioural management and lifestyle adaptation. Self-management can be delivered in groups or on an individual basis and can be generic or disease specific. The occupational therapist can facilitate a self-management approach by supporting the person living with a long-term neurological condition to (Schulman-Green et al., 2012):

Take ownership of their health needs
- Access accurate and up-to-date information about the condition
- Monitor and manage symptoms
- Recognise limitations
- Adjust routines to manage symptoms and side effects
- Attend regular medical reviews
- Manage medication
- Manage symptoms, for example fatigue management and pain management

Become an expert
- Set realistic goals
- Share decision-making
- Develop problem-solving skills
- Plan, prioritising and pace
- Develop confidence and self-efficacy

Engage in health promoting activities
- Exercise
- Nutrition and diet
- Smoking cessation
- Alcohol reduction
- Reduce stress
- Maintain life-style changes

Process emotions
- Grieve, explore and express emotional responses
- Deal with shock of diagnosis, self-blame and guilt

Adjustment
- Make sense of illness
- Identify and confront change and loss, for example changes in physical function, role, identity, body image, control and mortality
- Manage uncertainty
- Develop coping strategies
- Deal with setbacks
- Focus on possibilities
- Accept the 'new normal'
- Clarify and re-establish roles
- Examine health beliefs
- Make social comparisons
- Choose who and when to disclose illness
- Deal with stigma

Integrate illness into daily life
- Reorganise everyday life
- Seek/obtain assistance
- Create consistent routines
- Control environment
- Be flexible
- Carry out normal tasks and responsibilities as much as possible
- Manage disruptions in school, work, family and social activities
- Balance living life with health needs
- Find new enjoyable activities

Meaning making
- Reflect on/rearrange priorities and values
- Reframe expectations of life and self
- Come to terms with terminal condition and end of life
- Learn personal strengths and limitations
- Become empowered
- Be altruistic, that is unselfish, humane and selfless
- Find meaning in work, relationships, activities and spirituality
- Create a sense of purpose
- Appreciate life

3.5 Co-production

Co-production is an approach which recognises the expertise of the person living with a long-term neurological condition in the design and delivery of services. Recent high-profile investigations, including the Francis Report (Francis, 2010), highlighted the need for the development of more equal partnerships between care providers and people who use services, their families and carers (Social Care Institute for Excellence [SCIE], 2013). Co-production offers a concept and a framework to develop these more meaningful relationships (SCIE, 2013).

Co-production facilitates occupational therapists and people living with a long-term neurological condition 'to make better use of each other's assets, resources and contributions to achieve better outcomes or improved efficiency' (Bovaird and Löeffler, 2012). The key features of co-production include the following:
- Breaking down barriers between people who use services and professionals
- Building on people's existing capabilities
- Reciprocity, where people get something back for having done something for others
- Mutuality through people working together to achieve their shared interests
- Working with peer and personal support networks alongside professional networks
- Facilitating services by helping organisations to become agents for change rather than just being service providers (SCIE, 2013).

Co-production differs from self-management in that people living with a long-term neurological condition become involved in the design and organisation of services within their communities in an equal and reciprocal relationship with the occupational therapist. Co-production differs from participation which involves consultation with people living with a long-term neurological condition while co-production would view them as equal partners and co-creators (SCIE, 2012). Within a co-creative model people living with a long-term neurological condition would contribute to the design and delivery of services while co-production would require people living with a long-term neurological condition to take on some of the work done by the occupational therapist (Cottam and Leadbetter, 2004).

Transformative co-production is about:

- Occupational therapists and people living with a long-term neurological condition working as equal partners towards shared goals
- Moving from involvement and participation towards people living with a long-term neurological condition, their families and carers having an equal, more meaningful and more powerful role in services
- Involving people living with a long-term neurological condition in all aspects of a service including planning, development and actual delivery of the service
- Transferring power and resources to people living with a long-term neurological condition, their families and carers
- Valuing the strengths and assets of people living with a long-term neurological condition
- Recognising that if someone makes a contribution they should get something back in exchange.

3.6 Evaluating your practice

Person-centred models of care are often seen to be at odds with evidence-based practice, yet the fundamental aim of person-centred care is to deliver a high quality of care and enhance client satisfaction (Sidani et al., 2006). Occupational therapists are becoming increasingly aware of the need to consider the importance of, and how they can contribute to, a positive client experience. Measurement of client experience requires a different approach from that of measuring satisfaction. While client satisfaction seeks to identify how the individual's care fulfilled their expectations, client experience focuses on how the care experience made the person feel.

Patient experience is increasingly recognised as one of the three pillars of quality in healthcare alongside clinical effectiveness and patient safety (Institute of Medicine, 2001b). Measuring client experience provides key information on the interaction between the person living with a long-term neurological condition and the occupational therapist. Key aspects of measuring patient experience include (Doyle et al., 2013) the following:

- Empathy
- Respecting preferences

- Involvement in decision-making
- Enabling and empowering
- Respect
- Dignity
- Compassion
- Kindness
- Understanding values, beliefs and choices
- Clear, comprehensible information and communications
- Effective care delivered by trusted professionals
- Timely, tailored and expert management
- Attention to the physical environment, that is safety and comfort
- Co-ordination, continuity and smooth transition of care.

3.6.1 Measures of client experience

The following client experience questionnaires are available for use by occupational therapists:

- **The Consultation and Relational Empathy (CARE)** is a patient-assessed measure designed for use in the clinical setting to evaluate the quality of the consultation in terms of the 'human' aspects of care. Although the CARE measure is validated for occupational therapists working in secondary care, it is not feasible for use within in-patient settings or for occupational therapists involved in the care of a small number of clients. The 10-item questionnaire can be completed by people living with a long-term neurological condition following a consultation with the occupational therapist using a five point rating scale from 'poor' to 'excellent' (Mercer et al., 2004).
- **The PPE-15** is a patient experience questionnaire designed for use in inpatient care settings (Jenkinson et al., 2002). It is a short version of the Picker Adult In-Patient Questionnaire Picker, developed by the Picker Institute. This 15-item questionnaire can be used by occupational therapists to evaluate specific healthcare processes that impact on quality using a scoring system of four possible answers based on yes/no response categories.
- **Patient Experience Questionnaire (PEQ)** developed by Steine et al. (2001) was designed for use in primary health care for measuring patient experience in the domains of interaction, emotion and consultation outcome. The questionnaire includes 18 items in five dimensions: communication, emotions, short-term outcome, barriers and relations with auxiliary staff.

3.7 Self-evaluation questions

1 What are the underlying principles of person-centred care?
2 What are the benefits of person-centred care to the client?
3 What are the benefits of person-centred care to the occupational therapist?

4 What are the six key stages of person-centred care?

5 What are the five elements of client-centred practice?

6 What skills are required for delivering client-centred practice?

7 What are the barriers to delivering client-centred practice?

8 What are the three core domains of self-management?

9 How does co-production differ from self-management and co-creation?

10 Why is it important to measure client experience?

References

Barlow JH (2001) How to use education as an intervention in osteoarthritis. Best Practice & Research Clinical Rheumatology, 15(4):545–558.

Barlow J, Wright C, Sheasby J, Turner A and Hainsworth J (2002) Self-management approaches for people with chronic conditions: a review. Patient Education and Counseling, 48:177–187.

Bolmsjö I (2001) Existential issues in palliative care: interviews of patients with amyotrophic lateral sclerosis. Journal of Palliative Medicine, 4(4):499–505.

Bovaird T and Loeffler E (2012) From engagement to co-production: how users and communities contribute to public services. In Brandsen T and Pestoff V (Eds) New public governance, the third sector and co-production. London: Routledge.

Canadian Association of Occupational Therapists (CAOT) and Department of National Health and Welfare (1983). Guidelines for the client-centred practice of occupational therapy (H39-33/1983E). Ottawa, ON: Department of National Health and Welfare.

Cottam H and Leadbetter C (2004) Health: co-creating services (Red Paper 01). London: Design Council.

Davis J, Craik J and Polatajko H (2007) Using the Canadian Process Practice Framework: amplifying the process. In Townsend E and Polatajko H (Eds) Enabling occupation 11: advancing an occupational therapy vision for health, well-being and justice through occupation. Ottawa, ON: CAOT Publications ACE, pp. 247–272.

Doyle C, Lennox L and Bell D (2013) A systematic review of evidence on the links between patient experience and clinical safety and effectiveness. BMJ Open, 3:e001570. doi:10.1136/bmjopen-2012-001570. Available at http://bmjopen.bmj.com/content/3/1/e001570.full (Accessed 31 October 2015).

Finset A (2011) Research on person-centred clinical care. Journal of Evaluation in Clinical Practice, 17:384–386.

Francis R (2010) Independent inquiry into care provided by Mid Staffordshire NHS Foundation Trust January 2005 – March 2009. London: HMSO.

Hagedorn R (1997) The occupational therapy process. In Hagedorn R (Ed.) Foundations for practice in occupational therapy, 2nd Edition. London: Churchill Livingstone Elsevier, pp. 9–15.

Howie JGR, Heaney D and Maxwell M (2004) Quality, core values and the general practice consultation: issues of definition, measurement and delivery. Family Practice, 21:458–468.

Institute of Medicine (2001a) *Envisioning the national health care quality report.* Available from http://www.nap.edu/catalog/10073/envisioning-the-national-health-care-quality-report (Accessed 3 April 2015).

Institute of Medicine (2001b) Crossing the quality chasm: a new health system for the 21st century. Washington, DC: National Academy Press.

Jenkinson C, Coulter A and Bruster S (2002) The Picker Patient Experience Questionnaire: development and validation using data from in-patient surveys in five countries. International Journal for Quality in Health Care, 14(5):353–358.

Kaplan RM (1991) Health-related quality of life in patient decision making. Journal of Social Sciences, 47:69–90.

Kennedy I (2003) Patients are experts in their own field. BMJ, 326:1276.

Law M, Baptiste S, McColl M, Opzoomer A, Polatajko H and Pollock N (1990) The Canadian occupational performance measure: an outcome measure for occupational therapy. Canadian Journal of Occupational Therapy [Revue Canadienne d Ergotherapie], 57(2):82–87.

Law M, Baptiste S and Mills J (1995) Client-centred practice: what does it mean and does it make a difference? Canadian Journal of Occupational Therapy, 62(5):250–257.

Lutz BJ and Bowers BJ (2000) Patient-centred care: understanding its interpretation and implementation in health care. Scholarly Inquiry for Nursing Practice, 14(2):165–183; discussion 183–187.

Malec JF (1999) Goal attainment scaling in rehabilitation. Neuropsychological Rehabilitation, 3/4(9):253–275.

Mead N and Bower P (2000) Patient-centredness: a conceptual framework and review of the empirical literature. Social Science and Medicine, 51:1087–1110.

Mercer S, Maxwell M, Heaney D and Watt G (2004) The consultation and relational empathy (CARE) measure: development and preliminary validation and reliability of an empathy-based consultation process measure. Family Practice, 21(6):699–705.

Morgan A (2002) Beginning to use a narrative approach in therapy. The International Journal of Narrative Therapy and Community Work, 2002(1):85–90.

National Institute for Health and Care Excellence (NICE) (2007) Behaviour change: the principles for effective interventions. NICE public health guidance 6. London: National Institute for Health and Care Excellence.

Neighbour R (1987) The inner consultation. Lancaster: MTP Press.

Oliver M (1996) Understanding disability: from theory to practice. Basingstoke: Macmillan.

Parkinson S, Forsyth K and Kielhofner G (2006) The Model of Human Occupation Screening Tool (MOHOST) Version 2.0. University of Illinois Board of Trustees. Available at http://www.cade.uic.edu/moho/products.aspx (Accessed 27 October 2015).

Person Centred Health and Care Collaborative (2014) People at the centre of health and care. Person Centred Health and Care Collaborative. Glasgow: Healthcare Improvement Scotland.

Picking C (2000) Working in partnership with disabled people. New perspectives for professionals within the social model of disability. In Cooper J (Ed.) Law, rights and disability. London: Kingsley, pp. 11–31.

Polatajko HJ, Davis JA and McEwen SE (2015) Therapeutic use of self: a catalyst in the client-therapist alliance for change. In Christiansen C, Baum C and Bass J (Eds) Occupational therapy: performance, participation and well-being, 4th Edition. Thorofare, NJ: Slack Incorporated, pp 81–92.

Ponte PR, Conlin G, Conway JB, Grant S, Medeiros C, Nies J, Shulman L, Branowicki P and Conley K (2003) Making patient-centred care come alive. JONA, 33(2):82–90.

Preston J, Haslam S and Lamont L (2012) What do people with multiple sclerosis want from an occupational therapy service? British Journal of Occupational Therapy, 75(6):264–270.

Preston J, Hammersley R and Gallagher H (2013) The executive dysfunctions most commonly associated with multiple sclerosis and their impact on occupational performance. British Journal of Occupational Therapy, 76(5):225–233.

Robinson JH, Callister LC, Berry JA and Dearing KA (2008) Patient-centred care and adherence: definitions and applications to improve outcomes. Journal of the American Academy of Nurse Practitioners, 20:600–607.

Schulman-Green D, Jaser S, Martin F, Alonzo A, Grey M, McCorkle R, Redeker NS, Reynolds N and Whittemore R (2012) Processes of self-management in chronic illness. Journal of Nursing Scholarship, 44(2):136–144.

Schulz R and Heckhausen J (1996) A life span model of successful aging. American Psychologist, 51:702–714.

Shakespeare T and Watson N (2002) The social model of disability: an outdated ideaology? Research in Social Science and Disability, 2:9–28.

Shaw V (2001) Needs first: a good practice guide for RSL's to prioritise tenants' needs for adaptations. York: HoDis (National Disabled Persons Housing Services Ltd).

Sidani S, Epstein D and Miranda J (2006) Eliciting patient treatment preferences: a strategy to integrate evidence-based and patient-centred care. Worldviews on Evidence-Based Nursing, 3(3):116–123.

Siegert RJ, McPherson KM and Taylor WJ (2004) Towards a cognitive-affective model of goal-setting in rehabilitation: is self-regulation theory a key step? Disability and Rehabilitation, 26(20):1175–1183.

Social Care Institute for Excellence (SCIE) (2012) Towards co-production: taking participation to the next level, SCIE Report 53. London: SCIE.

Social Care Institute for Excellence (SCIE) (2013) Co-production in social care: what it is and how to do it. SCIE Guide 51. London: SCIE.

Steine S, Finset A and Laerum E (2001) A new, brief questionnaire (PEQ) developed in primary care for measuring patients' experience of health interaction, emotion and consultation outcome. Family Practice, 18(4):410–417.

Stewart M, Brown J, Weston W, McWhinney I, McMillan C and Freeman T (1995) Patient-centred medicine: transforming the clinical method. London: Sage.

Sumison T and Smyth G (2000) Barriers to client-centredness and their resolution. Canadian Journal of Occupational Therapy, 67(1):15–21.

The Health Foundation (2014) Person-centred care made simple: what everyone should know about person-centred care. London: The Health Foundation.

The Kings Fund (2011) Making shared decision making a reality: no decision about me, without me. London: The Kings Fund.

The Kings Fund (2012) Leadership and engagement for improvement in the NHS: together we can. London: The Kings Fund.

World Health Organisation (1986) Ottawa charter for health promotion. Ottawa, ON: Canadian Public Health Association, Health and Welfare Canada.

Wrosch C, Scheifer MF, Carver CS and Schulz R (2003) The importance of goal disengagement in adaptive self-regulation: when giving up is beneficial. Self and Identity, 2:1–20.

CHAPTER 4
Theoretical basis

4.1 Introduction

Neurological practice is a complex area of occupational therapy practice. Application of the underlying theoretical concepts of occupational therapy can at times seem challenging, particularly within the context of progressive neurological conditions. This chapter explores the relationship between occupational therapy knowledge and core skills and how they can be applied to neurological practice. The content of this chapter will be framed within the model developed by the College of Occupational Therapists (College of Occupational Therapists, 2014; Figure 4.1).

4.2 Definitions of occupational therapy

A number of definitions of occupational therapy have been developed over the years, but the definition which will be used within the context of this book is that of the College of Occupational Therapists (2009) as follows:

> Occupational therapists view people as occupational beings. People are intrinsically active and creative, needing to engage in a balanced range of activities in their daily lives in order to maintain health and wellbeing. People shape, and are shaped by, their experiences and interactions with their environments. They create identity and meaning through what they do and have the capacity to transform through pre-meditated and autonomous action.
>
> The purpose of occupational therapy is to enable people to fulfil, or to work towards fulfilling, their potential as occupational beings. Occupational therapists promote function, quality of life and the realisation of potential in people who are experiencing occupational deprivation, imbalance or alienation. They believe that activity can be an effective medium for remediating dysfunction, facilitating adaptation and recreating identity.

Occupational Therapy and Neurological Conditions, First Edition. Edited by Jenny Preston and Judi Edmans.
© 2016 John Wiley & Sons, Ltd. Published 2016 by John Wiley & Sons, Ltd.

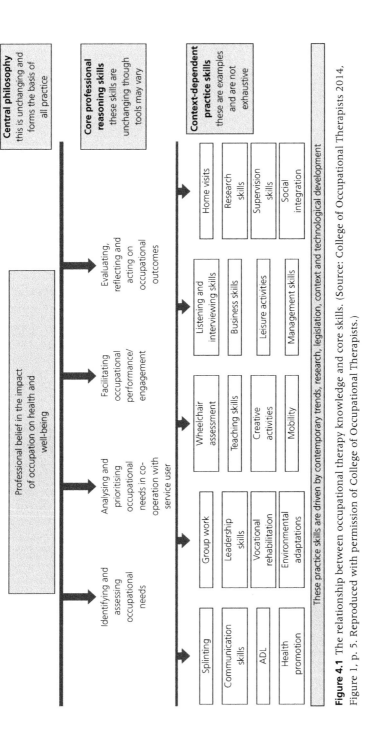

Figure 4.1 The relationship between occupational therapy knowledge and core skills. (Source: College of Occupational Therapists 2014, Figure 1, p. 5. Reproduced with permission of College of Occupational Therapists.)

4.3 Central philosophy of occupational therapy

The central philosophy of occupational therapy forms the basis of all practice and is developed from the professional belief in the impact of occupation on health and wellbeing (College of Occupational Therapists, 2014). Health was originally defined by the World Health Organisation in 1948 as 'the state of complete physical, mental and social wellbeing and not merely the absence of disease or infirmity' and has remained unchanged since then. Reed (2015) challenges the ongoing use of this definition of health as a concept in occupational therapy and the assumption that 'occupation contributes positively to health' seeking further advancement of the understanding of the relationship between health and occupation from an occupational perspective.

Engagement in meaningful occupations is associated with positive physical health and longevity (Krause, 1991; Krause and Kjorsvig, 1992; Ville et al., 2001); contributes to perceptions of competence, capability, value and enhancing the quality of life itself (Hammell, 2004); and engagement in occupations with and for others generates a sense of belonging that is important to a sense of well-being (Hammell, 2004; Piškur et al., 2002; Waldie, 2002). Specific research involving people with multiple sclerosis (MS) (Reynolds and Prior, 2003) shows that envisioning a future engaged in meaningful occupations contributes to a sense of hope, which is identified as integral to positive well-being (Hammell, 2007).

4.4 Core professional reasoning skills

Working with people with long-term neurological conditions, like many other areas of occupational therapy practice, requires high-level thinking and reasoning skills (Bannigan and Moores, 2009). This can involve complex decision making with regards to the following:
• Identifying and assessing occupational needs
• Analysing and prioritising occupational needs in co-operation with the client
• Facilitating occupational performance and engagement
• Evaluating, reflecting and acting on occupational outcomes (College of Occupational Therapists, 2014).

Occupational therapists are required to draw on scientific knowledge in the form of evidence-based practice, yet there remain many areas in the management of long-term neurological conditions in which strong evidence about the efficacy of interventions is not yet available. In the absence of scientific evidence occupational therapists rely on 'best' clinical practice.

Professional thinking therefore involves a 'combination of deliberation, rational thinking, clinical reasoning, professional knowing and expertise gained from previous knowledge' (Donaghy and Morss, 2000). Critical reflection on one's practice and clinical reasoning skills can prepare an occupational therapist for all the years of practice as well as for lifelong learning and professional growth

(Leicht and Dickerson, 2001). Clinical reasoning may be developed with experience, but experience alone does not guarantee progression through the developmental sequence (Benamy, 1996; Slater and Cohn, 1991). Expert clinical reasoning is a vital skill for occupational therapists in today's rapidly changing health and social care environments and 'may be the strongest building block of the profession as it diversifies and grows to meet today's challenges' (Leicht and Dickerson, 2001).

4.4.1 Clinical reasoning

Clinical reasoning is defined as 'the thinking processes associated with conducting a clinical practice' (Unsworth, 2001). Clinical reasoning is the 'complex thought process occupational therapists use during all therapeutic interactions and is the main process used to integrate client assessment information and formulate an intervention plan' (Neistadt et al., 1998).

Clinical reasoning in occupational therapy practice has been found to differ from medical and nursing primarily due to the emphasis on the individual aspects of the client and their future occupational possibilities as opposed to the more immediate presenting medical problems (Leicht and Dickerson, 2001). Mattingly and Fleming (1994) acknowledged that occupational therapists focus on the meaning for the client, while the medical profession focuses on obtaining a diagnosis in order to cure disease and prevent death of the client (Leicht and Dickerson, 2001).

Furthermore occupational therapists are found to clinically reason throughout the treatment process and not solely at the assessment phase (Schell and Cervero, 1993). Occupational therapists engage in a range of forms of clinical reasoning which can include the following:

• Diagnostic reasoning
• Procedural reasoning
• Interactive reasoning
• Conditional reasoning
• Narrative reasoning
• Scientific reasoning
• Pragmatic reasoning
• Ethical reasoning.

Diagnostic reasoning is defined as a series of cognitive operations the occupational therapist performs to formulate the occupational therapy 'diagnosis'. This occurs within a two-phase process which focuses on problem identification and formulation of an intervention plan (Leicht and Dickerson, 2001). Key factors which support this process include the client's medical diagnosis, reason for referral, client's goals, targeted discharge environment, client's demographic characteristics, practice setting and the therapist's frame of reference (Rogers and Holm, 1997). The information obtained through this process is then used to formulate a hypothesis about occupational performance which can be refined and discarded as further information becomes available through relevant assessments and data collection. This pattern of occupational dysfunction is then compared to the occupational therapists prior knowledge and experience to inform a diagnostic statement or problem identification (Leicht and Dickerson, 2001).

Procedural reasoning places emphasis on the client's dysfunction and what procedures may alleviate the problem or remediate the client's functional performance problems (Mattingly and Fleming, 1994). In this form of reasoning the emphasis is on the 'process of defining the client's diagnostically related occupational performance area, performance component, and performance context problems, and selecting appropriate interventions' (Leicht and Dickerson, 2001). Fleming (1991a) views procedural reasoning in occupational therapy as the product of working within a medical model of care and compares this form of problem solving with the process of diagnosis, prognosis and prescription commonly used by physicians.

Interactive reasoning is used to help therapists interact and better understand the client (Leicht and Dickerson, 2001). Interactive reasoning leads to an understanding of what the disease or disability means to the client. Occupational therapists use interactive reasoning to develop an impression of the client as a person and his/her needs, interests and attitudes and then use this to obtain client collaboration in the therapy process and is used to experience the disability from the client's perspective (Leicht and Dickerson, 2001). Schwartz (1991) argues for a strong commitment to the caring perspective within occupational therapy, which is concerned predominantly with people and their relationships, in contrast to the justice perspective in which truth, justice and equality are the guiding principles. Occupational therapists emphasise the need for a strong therapeutic relationship for the therapeutic process to be successful (Mattingly, 1991a; Schwartz, 1991). Additionally occupational therapists 'use interactive reasoning to engage or motivate the client in the treatment session, and to match treatment goals and strategies with the client's interests and wishes. Interactive reasoning is also used to determine if the treatment session is going well and to construct a shared language for therapy between the therapist and the client' (Leicht and Dickerson, 2001). Interactive reasoning can also be used to convey a sense of trust, acceptance and hope to the client through the use of humour to relieve tension (Alnervik and Sviden, 1996; Fleming, 1991a).

Conditional reasoning is a 'complex form of social reasoning that is used to help the client participate in the difficult process of reconstructing his/her life after a permanent change due to an illness or injury' (Mattingly and Fleming, 1994). Conditional reasoning embodies the holistic perspective of the person's situation and is dependent on the participation of both the client and the therapist (Fleming, 1991a). Within this process occupational therapists need empathy and an ability to imagine how a client's condition could change using both current and future contexts, involving the client in the construction of an image of the possible outcome (Neistadt, 1998). Conditional reasoning is a complex multi-dimensional process that does not follow a strictly logical sequence, is not strictly cognitive, and is not always a conscious process (Fleming, 1991b; Mattingly and Fleming, 1994). In conditional reasoning the occupational therapist is attempting to integrate both the procedural and interactive reasoning components into one and then moving this focus onto the future of the client (Alnervik and Sviden, 1996; Fleming, 1991b).

Narrative reasoning is fundamental to occupational therapy as it 'seeks to make sense of the reality by linking the outside world to the inner world of intention and motivation' (Mattingly, 1991b). While the emphasis on the disease or diagnosis is fundamental in other models of reasoning the focus of narrative reasoning is undoubtedly on the client's experience of the disease and how that interacts with the person's life story (Mattingly, 1991b). The skill of the occupational therapist lies in the ability to 'put it all together' (Leicht and Dickerson, 2001). Narrative reasoning is central to the occupational therapy process and involves viewing therapy as a chapter in the client's life story. Narrative reasoning includes not only telling the retrospective life story but also involving the client in prospective story building (Leicht and Dickerson, 2001).

Scientific reasoning is one of four facets of clinical reasoning defined by Schell and Cervero (1993). Scientific reasoning is described as 'a framework for the understanding of the condition affecting the individual and determining the appropriate treatment interventions' (Schell, 1998). Diagnostic reasoning and procedural reasoning are considered the two forms of scientific reasoning (Schell, 1998).

Pragmatic reasoning is the second facet defined by Schell and Cervero (1993) and considers all practical issues that affect occupational therapy services, such as treatment environment; the therapists' values, knowledge, abilities and experiences; the client's social and financial resources; and the client's potential discharge environment (Neistadt, 1998). Pragmatic reasoning allows the therapist to decide what can be done for a particular client in a given treatment setting (Neistadt et al., 1998) and addresses the practical realities associated with service delivery in the present health and social care environments (Schell, 1998). While pragmatic reasoning is thought to have positive effects on the therapeutic process, overemphasis on pragmatic reasoning may not allow for individualisation (Leicht and Dickerson, 2001).

Ethical reasoning is strongly related to the therapists' values and as such has some parallels with Fleming's (1991b) ethical and moral decision-making. The emphasis within this facet is on the aspects of ethical reasoning by focussing not on 'what could be done' in a therapy session, but 'should be done' reflecting the competing challenges of service delivery, client preferences and possible treatment options (Leicht and Dickerson, 2001).

4.5 Conceptual models of occupational therapy practice

Occupational therapists rely on conceptual models of practice to provide the language and tools to help define the problems, develop effective interventions and evaluate the impact. The following key conceptual models of practice can be applied to neurological practice:
- Model of Human Occupation (MOHO)
- Canadian Model of Occupational Performance and Enablement (CMOP-E)
- The Person–Environment–Occupation–Performance (PEOP) model
- The Kawa (River) model
- The Occupational Model (Australia) (OPM-A)

4.5.1 Model of Human Occupation

The MOHO is defined as a 'client-centred, occupation-focussed, evidence-based conceptual model of practice which embraces the complexity of people's occupational needs' (Forsyth and Kielhofner, 2011). Within this model there is recognition that human occupation is complex, context-dependent and that occupations shape a person's self-perception and identity. Fundamental to the MOHO (Figure 4.2) are the concepts of :
- Volition: the motivation for occupation (including personal causation, values and interests)
- Habituation: the routine patterning of occupation (including habits and roles)
- Performance capacity: the nature of skilled performance (including physical environments, social and cultural contexts, motor, process, communication and interaction skills.

Figure 4.3 illustrates how MOHO can be applied.

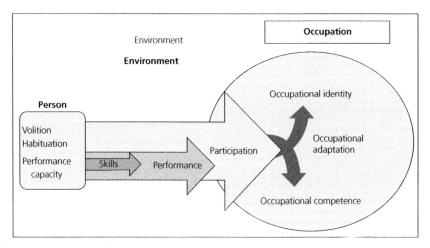

Figure 4.2 The Model of Human Occupation (MOHO). (Source: Christiansen et al. 2015, Figure 3-6, p. 35. Reproduced with permission of Slack Incorporated.)

Example of application to neurological practice

Thirty-eight-year-old David is a former architect who lives with his family in a remote location in a house which he designed and built. Prior to the diagnosis of Huntington's disease (HD), David was a high achiever, with extremely high expectations of his own performance which he achieved with ease. David was a keen sportsman and excelled in highly developed motor skills, including stamina and co-ordination. He was confident and self-assured and led a busy work and family life. David was extremely proud of his role as father to his two daughters aged 4 and 7 years.

Beyond work David was a professional singer. He was a very keen musician and enjoyed football. David thrived on his independence and control over his own life.

During the last 18 months, David has become symptomatic and is now experiencing difficulties due to involuntary movements, cognitive changes, low mood and reduced stamina. David is now dependent on others for everyday tasks.

4.5.2 Canadian Model of Occupational Performance and Enablement

Within this model, Townsend and Polatajko (2007) conceptualise occupational performance as the 'dynamic interaction of person, occupation, and environment'. The person is considered within the context of spiritual, physical, affective and cognitive components (Figure 4.4). Occupation is defined within self-care, productivity and leisure. This social model includes the cultural, physical and social environments encompassing the economic, legal and political environments. The physical environment provides a contextual model to identify barriers and enablers to participation, while the social environment reflects the importance of roles and relationships. The inclusion of the institutional environment incorporates factors which can contribute to the identification of occupational deprivation and occupational injustice. The main tool associated with this model, the Canadian Occupational Performance Measure (COPM) will also be discussed in Chapter 6.

Example of application to neurological practice

Linda is 41 years old and was diagnosed with Multiple Sclerosis 14 years ago. Linda is married with 2 children aged 6 years and 18 months. Linda's medical condition has developed a slowly progressive pattern over the time, allowing her to gradually adjust as changes occurred. Linda has good insight into her condition, is very positive and well-motivated, and is extremely focussed on her roles as a wife and mother. Table 4.1 illustrates how COPM can be applied to Linda.

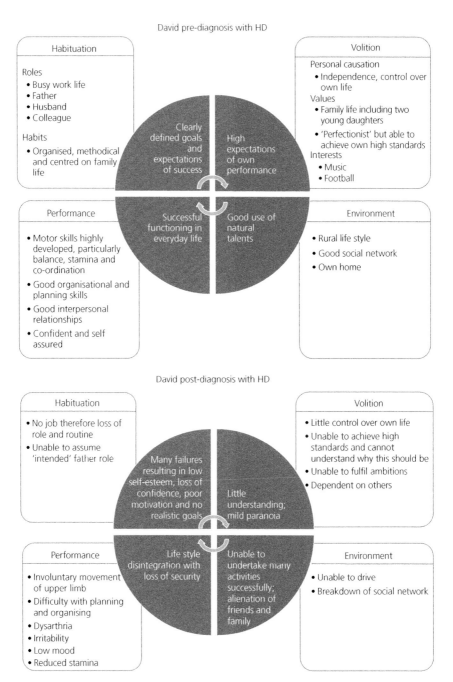

Figure 4.3 Illustration of MOHO applied to neurological practice.

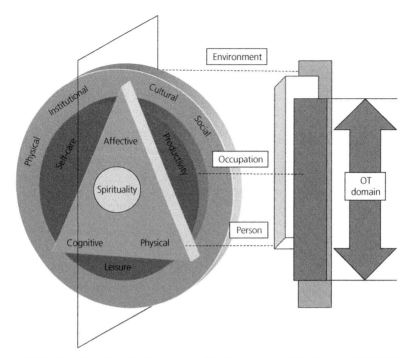

Figure 4.4 The Canadian Model of Occupational Performance and Enablement (CMOP-E). (Source: Turpin and Iwama 2011, Figure 5.1, p. 118. Reproduced with permission of Churchill Livingstone Elsevier, Toronto.)

Table 4.1 Practical example of COPM applied to neurological practice.

	Performance	Satisfaction	Importance
Self-care			
• Difficulties with prolonged standing in the kitchen	4	2	9
• Difficulties carrying and manipulating objects due to upper limb weakness and sensory impairment	5	4	9
• Difficulty standing in the shower	4	4	8
Leisure			
• Lack of opportunity for leisure activities	1	3	5
• Lack of stamina for leisure following demands of daily routine	1	2	7
Productivity			
• Problems with the impact of fatigue on all household tasks	2	4	5
• Difficulties participating in play with children	5	1	10
• Difficulty carrying baby due to upper limb weakness	3	1	10
• Difficulty manipulating small fastenings on children's clothes	4	2	9
• Difficulty remembering appointments	3	2	8

4.5.3 The Person-Environment-Occupational Performance (PEOP) model

Like many others this ecological-transactional systems model focuses on the characteristics of the person and his or her living environment recognising the dynamic and reciprocal interaction of the person, environment and occupational performance elements (Baum et al., 2015, p. 49; Christiansen et al., 2015; Figure 4.5). The PEOP model emphasises the client's perspective and facilitates the creation of a complete occupational profile including the client's perception of the current situation and includes consideration of roles, interests, responsibilities and/or mission and values (Christiansen et al., 2011). This model bridges biomedical and socio-cultural models within three relevant domains of knowledge for occupational therapy practice: person factors, environmental factors and occupations (Christiansen et al., 2011). The PEOP model supports client-centred practice, in that it values and requires the input of the individual to define the context, identify resources and formulate important goals (Christiansen et al., 2011).

Example of application to neurological practice

Lewis is 34 years old. Both he and his wife were eagerly awaiting the birth of their first child when Lewis was diagnosed with MND. Previously Lewis worked full time as a storeman. Tables 4.2 and 4.3 illustrate how PEOP can be applied to Lewis.

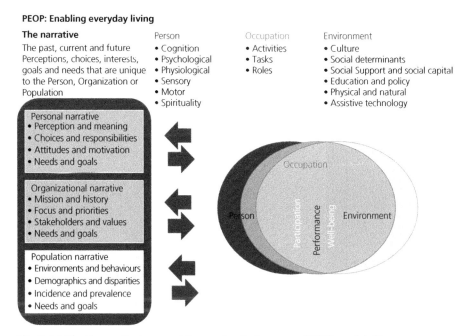

Figure 4.5 The Person-Environment-Occupation Performance (PEOP) model. (Source: Christiansen et al. 2015, Figure 3-9, p. 39. Reproduced with permission of Slack Incorporated.)

Table 4.2 Practical application of PEOP person factors to neurological practice.

Person factors

Motor	Sensory	Physiological	Cognition	Psychological	Meaning, sense making and spirituality
Includes abnormal synergy, associated movement, athetosis, balance, bradykinesia, chorea, coordination, blocked practice, distributed practice, dysdiadochokinesthesia, extrinsic or augmented feedback, hypermetria	Includes audition, detection, discrimination, gustatory, multi-sensory, olfactory, perception, proprioception, recognition, sensory processing	Includes aerobic physical activity, body composition, body mass, bone-strength, cardiac endurance, flexibility, general health, muscle endurance, muscle endurance, nutritional status	Includes attention, awareness/insight, cognitive function, communication, executive function, learning, memory, social awareness	Includes affect, coping, emotional regulation, identity, life balance, mood, motivation, self-concept, self-efficacy, self-esteem, well-being	Includes meaning, mind–body connections, motivation, personal life stories, personal well-being
• Muscle weakness • Loss of power • Dysarthria • Fasciculation	• Neuropathic pain • Excessive salivation • Runny nose	• Respiratory insufficiency • Fatigue • Pre-existing type 1 diabetes • Weight loss due to swallowing difficulties	• Cognitively intact	• Low mood • Withdrawn • Dependency on others • Little control over his own life • Unable to achieve previous high standards • Loss of roles • Loss of routine • Loss of confidence • Loss of self-esteem	• Difficulty understanding why he has been diagnosed with MND • Feels diagnosis is a punishment for a former life • Difficulty reconciling forward planning with new baby and his own life-limiting condition

Source: Adapted from: Christiansen C and Baum C (Eds) Enabling Function and Well-Being, Figure 3-7, p. 62. Reproduced with permission of Baum C.

Table 4.3 Practical application of PEOP performance enablers and components to neurological practice.

Intrinsic performance enablers and corresponding performance components

Culture	Social determinants of health, social capital and social support	Physical and natural environment	Health, education, social and public policies	Technology
Includes beliefs, values, customs, power, decision-making	Includes health inequalities, social capital, social connectedness, social support, social cohesion	Includes the built environment, natural environment, physical environment	Includes advocacy, equality, healthcare utilisation, occupational justice, social justice	Includes accessible design, assistive technology, digital technology, context, device discontinuance, ergonomics
• Dominant male role	• Intimate family group, does not involve extended family	• Lives in private home with bedroom and bathroom upstairs	• Does not engage with healthcare services as has difficulty accepting diagnosis	• Using tablet device for social media
• Breadwinner	• Does not engage in local community	• Home is situated at the top of a hill	• Not eligible for provision of stair lift at home due to Local Authority criteria	• Awaiting environmental control system to be installed to reduce reliance on his wife
• Expectations of forthcoming fatherly role	• Close working and personal relationship with a 'selected few' at work	• Work environment includes heavy machinery	• Unable to continue in work due to inability to put reasonable adjustments in place due to progressive nature of his medical condition	• Uses non-invasive ventilation at night
• Not willing to accept support	• Lives in rural community with lack of public transport	• Work base is 30-minute drive from home		• PEG tube inserted due to swallowing difficulties
• Very private person	• Disengaged from social activities	• Wheelchair doesn't fit in family car along with the pram		• Uses riser/recliner chair
• Previously very independent				

Source: Adapted from: Christiansen C and Baum 1997 in Christiansen C and Baum C (Eds) Enabling function and well-being, Figure 3-6, p. 60. Reproduced with permission of Baum C.

4.5.4 The Kawa (River) model

This model was developed from a foundation that each person's experience of and meanings they attach to daily life are unique (Lim and Iwama, 2006; Turpin and Iwama (2011); Figure 4.6). Conceptually developed through the metaphor of a river clients are facilitated to portray an image of their 'personal river' to symbolise their life journey. Aspects of the environment such as rocks (to reflect life circumstances), walls and bottom (signifying environmental factors) and driftwood (representing assets and liabilities) are creatively used to enable life flow. Stages of the river reflect the personal life journey including the past, present and future with personal health and wellbeing expressed by a free and unrestricted flow of one's river. This model reflects a departure from the more traditional models which are often interpreted and applied at an impairment level in practice.

Example of application to neurological practice

Bill is 64 years old and was diagnosed with the progressive muscular atrophy (PMA) form of motor neurone disease (MND). There is a family history of MND as Bill witnessed both his father and his uncle progress through their personal journeys with the disease. Bill is fully aware of what lies ahead for him but feels that the slower rate of progression gives him more time to prepare for his own journey with MND. Using the Kawa (River) model to facilitate narrative discussion the occupational therapist developed a more holistic understanding of Bill's current needs and how occupational therapy can support change within his particular life circumstances.

Water (representing life flow): Bill indicated that his personal river was flowing freely at this stage. Bill reflected on the diagnosis of MND as providing him with an opportunity to cleanse and renew his spirit, casting aside aspects of bitterness and regret which had previously dominated his being. Bill felt that having a diagnosis with a life-limiting condition allowed him to free his mind and spirit of unnecessary burden, anger and disappointment in both himself and others and allowed him to re-prioritise all aspects of his life. Bill now feels more in touch with his purpose in life and feels a sense of freedom to allow his river to flow naturally and peacefully towards its eventual destination.

River walls and river floor: Bill believes that his river is very firmly contained within a strong social and physical environment. Bill feels particularly well supported within a very close family dynamic and believes that the previous experience of his father and uncle facilitates an openness and honesty in their preparations for his final journey.

Rocks: The ongoing physical changes and deterioration are represented by Bill's rocks. Bill is aware of a reduction in function in his upper limbs, reduced mobility, difficulty standing and fatigue.

Driftwood: Bill has considerable insight into his situation which facilitates an inner strength and positivity which is undoubtedly helping Bill to cope. Bill is content with his achievements in life and feels that he has provided sufficiently for his family who will continue to be well supported after his death. Bill is an extrovert, who thrives on being around family and friends. He loves to be the centre of attention and always has a story to tell.

Space: Bill's goals were not developed around the removal of obstructions within his river but instead to facilitate his river to continue to flow freely. This included timely provision of equipment to allow him to maintain his independence.

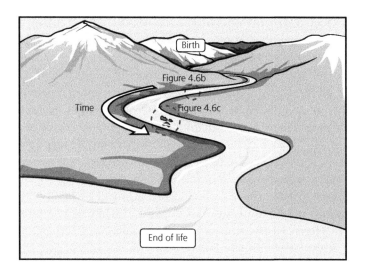

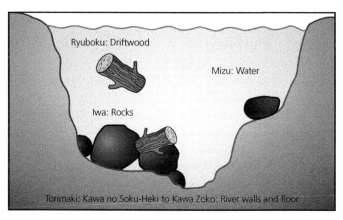

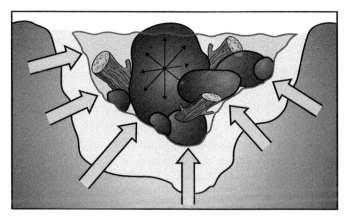

Figure 4.6 The Kawa (River) model; (a) The river; (b) Elements of the river; (c) Elements constricting water flow. (Source: Turpin and Iwama 2011, Figures 7.1–7.3, pp. 160–161. Reproduced with permission of Churchill Livingstone Elsevier.)

4.5.5 The Occupational Performance Model (Australia) OPM-A

The underlying assumptions of this model also reflect the life-long relationship between the person and their environment and the dynamic interaction through occupation. The theoretical structure incorporates eight major constructs: occupational performance; occupational performance roles; occupational performance areas (rest, self-maintenance, productivity, leisure); components of occupational performance (biomechanical, sensory-motor, cognitive, intrapersonal, interpersonal); core elements of occupational performance (body, mind, spirit); environment (physical, sensory, cultural, social); and space and time with each item incorporating many interrelating elements (Chapparo and Ranka, 1997). The main tool developed for use with this model is The Perceive, Recall, Plan and Perform (PRPP) System of Task Analysis (Chapparo and Ranka, 1997). This criterion-referenced assessment has been developed as an ecological measure designed to assess task-embedded information processing capacity during occupational therapy assessment.

4.6 Frames of reference

The conceptual models previously described have been developed from within the profession specifically to inform occupational therapy practice. However occupational therapists also utilise frames of reference developed outside the profession which, if used appropriately, can be applied within occupational therapy practice (Duncan, 2011). The frames of reference which are most commonly accessed within neurological practice include the following:
• The Cognitive Behavioural Frame of Reference
• The Biomechanical Frame of Reference
• The Neurodevelopmental Approach.
   Each frame of reference will now be considered in relation to long-term neurological conditions.

4.6.1 Cognitive Behavioural Frame of Reference

The Cognitive Behavioural Frame of Reference is an approach developed within the psychological therapies and includes a range of techniques such as behavioural modification and cognitive behavioural therapy (CBT). Increasingly occupational therapists are utilising a cognitive behavioural approach within their practice, particularly within mental health services (Duncan, 2011).

   Within a cognitive behavioural approach the underlying assumption is that distorted or unrealistic thoughts or irrational fears can impact on a person's ability to function successfully within their everyday routines. An example of this might be where a person diagnosed with a long-term neurological condition experiences depression. Recent evidence has confirmed that depression in long-term neurological conditions has been associated with breakdowns in personal relationships and employment, cognitive impairment and decreased medication adherence leading to a heightened suicide risk and is recognised as a major determinant of quality of life (Hind et al., 2014).

Through the use of strategies including role play, facilitated groups and graded activity scheduling, the person is facilitated to challenge their underlying thoughts and beliefs turning maladaptive behavioural responses into adaptive behaviours which is reinforced through feelings of self-efficacy and improved outcomes in everyday tasks and activities (Duncan, 2011).

Example of application to neurological practice

Christine is 54 years old and was diagnosed with Parkinson's 4 years ago. She experiences particular difficulties due to fatigue and the occupational therapist felt that Christine would benefit from participating in a fatigue management programme. Christine was extremely anxious and did not feel able to participate in a fatigue management programme as she worried that if she left the house that she might become unwell and that she not be able to get back home safely. A cognitive behavioural approach was used to support Christine to work through her fears about leaving her home, challenging her negative thoughts and turning them into positive behaviours.

Christine was supported through a graded exposure programme which initially started with her stepping outside her front door. Gradually she was encouraged to walk to the end of her garden path, then to the end of the street and so forth until she was confident enough to leave her home. Christine now attends a fatigue management group and benefits significantly from the peer support of other group members.

4.6.2 Biomechanical Frame of Reference

The Biomechanical Frame of Reference aims specifically to address the quality of movement in occupations (McMillan, 2011). The specific objectives of the biomechanical approach are to:

- Prevent deterioration and maintain existing movement for occupational performance
- Restore movement for occupational performance
- Compensate/adapt for loss of movement in occupational performance.

There is some debate as to whether the biomechanical frame of reference can be applied to neurological conditions; however, McMillan (2011) suggests there is some value in accessing the biomechanical approach to prevent shortening of soft tissue such as muscle tissue, connective tissue, tendons and ligaments.

Example of application to neurological practice

An example of where an occupational therapist used a biomechanical approach in clinical practice was with Claire who had been diagnosed with motor neurone disease 6 months earlier. When the occupational therapist met Claire she was still quite independent within her daily routines. She was however challenged by problems in her left (non-dominant) hand due to loss of power and strength. They discussed how this impacted on Claire's daily routines and at the time Claire was managing in an adapted way with her right hand. Claire identified that her left hand was 'getting in the way of her daily activities' due to the lack of movement in her fingers and wrist. They talked about why this was happening and that the damage which was occurring within her brain was irreversible and the function could not be restored. Claire also indicated that she was experiencing pain in her wrist. They discussed the possibility of splinting to support Claire's left hand to reduce the pain and to prevent further shortening of her muscles. Claire was fully aware that splinting would not promote recovery in her left hand.

4.6.3 Neurodevelopmental Frame of Reference

The key principles of the Neurodevelopmental Frame of Reference are based on motor control, neuromuscular facilitation and sensory integration. This approach requires an in-depth understanding of how the central nervous system processes sensory and perceptual information to produce controlled movement (Feaver and Ezekiel, 2011). The motor control frame of reference is more commonly associated with stroke rehabilitation through specific approaches including normal movement theory (Bobath, 1990) and motor relearning (Carr and Shepherd, 1987).

The key difference between stroke rehabilitation and the management of long-term neurological conditions relates to neuroplasticity, more commonly recognised as regeneration or repair of the brain following injury. In progressive neurological conditions this is less likely to occur although there is acknowledgement that recovery occurs between relapses in conditions like MS. The evidence base for the application of the neurodevelopmental frame of reference to long-term neurological conditions is not nearly as advanced as it is in relation to stroke.

Example of application to neurological practice

Michelle is 27 years old and was diagnosed with MS 2 years ago. Michelle's main difficulties relate to her mobility due to foot drop. Michelle has been fitted for an ankle-foot orthosis (AFO) which she wears with casual shoes and trousers. Michelle is currently planning her wedding and her goal is to be able to walk down the aisle wearing more 'glamorous' shoes with a low heel. Michelle has been trialling functional electrical stimulation (FES) which activates the dorsiflexors to improve walking speed and restore normal range of movement, subsequently allowing her to walk more confidently.

4.7 Context-dependent practice skills

4.7.1 Occupational therapy core skills

Core skills are described as the 'expert knowledge and abilities that are shared by all occupational therapists irrespective of their field or level of practice' (Creek, 2003). The College of Occupational Therapists (2009) outlined seven core skills as follows:

1 Collaboration with the client: building a collaborative relationship with the client that will promote reflection, autonomy and engagement in the therapeutic process

2 Assessment: assessing and observing functional potential, limitations, ability and needs, including the effects of physical and psychosocial environments

3 Enablement: enabling people to explore, achieve and maintain balance in their activities of daily living in the areas of personal care, domestic, leisure and (productive activities)

4 Problem solving: identifying and solving occupational performance problems

5 Using activity as a therapeutic tool: using activities to promote health, wellbeing and function by analysing, selecting, synthesising, adapting, grading and applying activities for specific therapeutic purposes

6 Group work: planning, organising and leading activity groups

7 Environmental adaptation: analysing and adapting environments to increase function and social participation.

4.7.2 Core values for neurological practice

In addition to the core skills occupational therapists are also required to demonstrate professionalism through their behaviour and values. Unlike the core skills which are shared across all areas of occupational therapy practice, Misch (2002) argues that the values of a profession within one environment may not be identified as relevant within another. However in order for occupational therapists working within neurological practice to uphold the professional values, it is imperative that those values are made explicit. The values adopted by the College of Occupational Therapists Specialist Section – Neurological Practice are those developed from a recent Australian study (Aguilar et al., 2012; Table 4.4).

4.7.3 Context-dependent practice skills for neurological practice

Within the College of Occupational Therapists (2014) model it is acknowledged that practice skills are context dependent and will be driven by contemporary trends, research, legislation, context and technological development. The following list of technical and cognitive skills has been developed by the College of Occupational Therapists Specialist Section – Neurological Practice as being indicative of the current requirements:

Technical skills

ADL	Anger management	Anxiety management
Assistive technology	Cognitive rehabilitation	Creative abilities
Driving	Environmental adaptations	Fatigue management
Home visits	Leisure	Managing challenging behaviours
Mindfulness	Motivational interviewing	Mobility
Mood management	Moving and handling	Perception
Postural management	Pressure care	Sleep management
Splinting	Vocational rehabilitation	Wheelchair assessment

Cognitive skills

Business skills	Communication skills	Counselling skills
Health promoting	Goal-setting skills	Leadership
Management	Outcome measurement	Research skills
Safeguarding mental capacity	Supervision	Teaching

Table 4.4 Core values for neurological practice.

Categories	Values
The client and the client–therapist partnership	Working with clients
	Empowering clients to lead
	Understanding the individual client
	Honouring client's priorities and goals
	Client independence
Occupational therapy knowledge, skills and practice	Using and updating knowledge and clinical skills
	Occupation
	Problem solving
	Self-reflection
	Working within a team
	Leadership within the workplace
	Advocacy
	Being a professional
Selfless values	Kindness
	Warmth
	Empathy
	Honesty
	Fairness
	Caring
	Thoughtfulness
	Humility
	Helping clients
	Giving hope
	Perseverance
	Respect

Source: Aguilar et al. 2012, Table 1, p. 211. Reproduced with permission of John Wiley & Sons.

4.8 Self-evaluation questions

1 What is the central philosophy of occupational therapy?
2 What are the four components of complex decision-making?
3 What are the four main forms of clinical reasoning accessed by occupational therapists?
4 Which form of clinical reasoning is most appropriate for occupational therapists working with people with long-term neurological conditions?
5 How does clinical reasoning in occupational therapy differ from medicine and nursing?
6 How do occupational therapists use conceptual models of practice?
7 What are the key conceptual models of practice which can be applied to people with neurological conditions?
8 What is the difference between conceptual models of practice and frames of reference?
9 Which frames of reference are most commonly applied to neurological practice?
10 Name at least three theoretical models of occupational therapy practice which can be applied to people with long-term neurological conditions.

References

Aguilar A, Stupans I, Scutter S and King S (2012) Exploring professionalism: the professional values of Australian occupational therapists. Australian Occupational Therapy Journal, 59:209–217.

Alnervik A and Sviden G (1996) On clinical reasoning: patterns of reflection on practice. The Occupational Therapy Journal of Research, 16:110.

Bannigan K and Moores A (2009) A model of professional thinking: integrating reflective practice and evidence based practice. Canadian Journal of Occupational Therapy, 75(5):342–350.

Baum C, Christiansen CH and Bass J (2015) The Person-Environment-Occupation-Performance (PEOP) model. In Christiansen C, Baum C and Bass J (Eds) Occupational therapy: performance, participation and well-being, 4th Edition. Thorofare, NJ: Slack Incorporated, pp. 49–55.

Benamy BC (1996) Developing clinical reasoning skills: strategies for occupational therapists. San Antonio, TX: Therapy Skill Builders.

Bobath B (1990) Adult hemiplegia evaluation and treatment. Oxford: Heinnemann Medical.

Carr JH and Shepherd RB (1987) A motor relearning programme for stroke, 2nd Edition. London: Heinnemann.

Chapparo C and Ranka J (1997) OPM: Occupational Performance Model (Australia), monograph 1. Castle Hill, NSW: Occupational Performance Network.

Christiansen C and Baum C (1997) Person-environment occupational performance: a conceptual model for practice. In Christiansen C and Baum C (Eds) Enabling function and well-being. Thorofare, NJ: Slack Incorporated, pp. 46–71.

Christiansen C, Baum CM and Bass J (2011) The Person-Environment-Occupational Performance (PEOP) model. In Duncan EAS (Ed.) Foundations for practice in occupational therapy, 5th Edition. Edinburgh: Elsevier Churchill Livingstone, pp. 94–104.

Christiansen C, Baum C and Bass J (2015) Occupational therapy: performance, participation and well-being, 4th Edition. Thorofare, NJ: Slack Incorporated.

College of Occupational Therapists (2009) COT/BAOT briefing number 23: definitions and core skills for occupational therapy. London: College of Occupational Therapists.

College of Occupational Therapists (2014) Learning and development standards for pre-registration education. London: College of Occupational Therapists.

Creek J (2003) Occupational therapy defined as a complex intervention. London: College of Occupational Therapists.

Donaghy ME and Morss K (2000) Guided reflection: a framework to facilitate and assess reflective practice within the discipline of physiotherapy. Physiotherapy Theory and Practice, 16:3–14.

Duncan EAS (2011) An introduction to conceptual models of practice and frames of reference. In Duncan EAS (Ed.) Foundations for practice in occupational therapy, 5th Edition. Edinburgh: Elsevier Churchill Livingstone, pp. 43–48.

Feaver S and Ezekiel L (2011) Theoretical approaches to more control and cognitive-perceptual function. In Duncan EAS (Ed.) Foundations for practice in occupational therapy, 5th Edition. Edinburgh: Elsevier Churchill Livingstone, pp. 195–205.

Fleming M (1991a) Clinical reasoning in medicine compared with clinical reasoning in occupational therapy. American Journal of Occupational Therapy, 45:988–996.

Fleming M (1991b) The therapist with the three-track mind. American Journal of Occupational Therapy, 45:1007–1014.

Forsyth K and Kielhofner G (2011) The Model of Human Occupation: embracing the complexity of occupation by integrating theory into practice and practice into theory. In Duncan EAS (Ed.) Foundations for practice in occupational therapy, 5th Edition. Edinburgh: Elsevier Churchill Livingstone, pp. 51–80.

Hammell KW (2004) Dimensions of meaning in the occupations of daily life. Canadian Journal of Occupational Therapy, 71:296–305.

Hammell KW (2007) The experience of rehabilitation following spinal cord injury: a meta-synthesis of qualitative findings. Spinal Cord, 45:260–274.

Hind D, Cotter J, Thake A, Bradburn M, Cooper C, Isaac C and House A (2014) Cognitive behavioural therapy for the treatment of depression in people with multiple sclerosis: a systematic review and meta-analysis. BMC Psychiatry, 14:5. doi:10.1186/1471-244X-14-5.

Krause JS (1991) Survival following spinal cord injury: a fifteen-year prospective study. Rehabilitation Psychology, 36:89–98.

Krause JS and Kjorsvig JM (1992) Mortality after spinal cord injury: a four year prospective study. Archives of Physical Medicine and Rehabilitation, 73:558–563.

Leicht SB and Dickerson A (2001) Clinical reasoning, looking back. Occupational Therapy in Health Care, 14(3/4):105–130.

Lim KH and Iwama M (2006). Emerging models – an Asian perspective: the Kawa (River) model. In Duncan E (Ed.) Foundations for practice. Edinburgh: Elsevier.

Mattingly C (1991a) What is clinical reasoning? American Journal of Occupational Therapy, 45:979–986.

Mattingly C (1991b) The narrative nature of clinical reasoning. American Journal of Occupational Therapy, 45:998–1005.

Mattingly C and Fleming M (1994) Clinical reasoning: forms of inquiry in a therapeutic practice. Philadelphia, PA: F.A. Davis.

McMillan IR (2011) The biomechanical frame of reference in occupational therapy. In Duncan EAS (Ed.) Foundations for practice in occupational therapy, 5th Edition. Edinburgh: Elsevier Churchill Livingstone, pp. 179–193.

Misch D (2002) Evaluating physician's professionalism and humanism: the case for humanism 'connoisseurs'. Academic Medicine, 77:489–495.

Neistadt M (1998) Teaching clinical reasoning as a thinking frame. American Journal of Occupational Therapy, 52:221–229.

Neistadt M, Wright J and Mulligan S (1998) Clinical reasoning case studies as teaching tools. American Journal of Occupational Therapy, 52:125–132.

Piškur B, Kinebanian A and Josephsson S (2002) Occupation and wellbeing: a study of some Slovenian people's experiences of engagement in occupation in relation to well-being. Scandinavian Journal of Occupational Therapy, 9:63–70.

Reed KL (2015) Key occupational therapy concepts in the person-occupational-environment-performance model: their origin and historical use in the occupational therapy literature. In Christiansen C, Baum C and Bass J (Eds) Occupational therapy: performance, participation and well-being, 4th Edition. Thorofare, NJ: Slack Incorporated, pp. 565–648.

Reynolds F and Prior S (2003) 'Sticking jewels in your life': exploring women's strategies for negotiating an acceptable quality of life with multiple sclerosis. Qualitative Health Research, 13:1225–1251.

Rogers J and Holm M (1997) Diagnostic reasoning: the process of problem identification. In Christiansen C and Baum C (Eds) Occupational therapy: enabling function and well-being, 2nd Edition. Thorofare, NJ: Slack Incorporated, pp. 136–156.

Schell B (1998) Clinical reasoning: the basis of practice. In Neistadt M and Crepeau E (Eds) Willard and Spackman's occupational therapy, 9th Edition. Philadelphia, PA: Lippincott, Williams, & Wilkins, pp. 90–100.

Schell B and Cervero R (1993) Clinical reasoning in occupational therapy: an integrative review. American Journal of Occupational Therapy, 47:605–610.

Schwartz K (1991) Clinical reasoning and new ideas on intelligence: implications for teaching and learning. American Journal of Occupational Therapy, 45:1033–1037.

Slater D and Cohn E (1991) Staff development through analysis of practice. American Journal of Occupational Therapy, 45:1038–1044.

Townsend E and Polatajko HJ (2007) Enabling occupation II: advancing an occupational therapy vision for health, well-being and justice. Ottawa, ON: Canadian Association of Occupational Therapists (CAOT) Publications ACE.

Turpin M and Iwama MK (2011) Using occupational therapy models in practice: a field guide. Toronto, ON: Churchill Livingstone Elsevier, pp. 118 and 160–161.

Unsworth CA (2001) The clinical reasoning of novice and expert occupational therapists. Scandinavian Journal of Occupational Therapy, 8:163–173.

Ville I, Ravaud J-F and Tetrafigap Group (2001) Subjective well-being and severe motor impairments: the Tetrafigap survey on the long-term outcome of tetraplegic spinal cord injured persons. Social Science and Medicine, 52:369–384.

Waldie E (2002) Triumph of the challenged: conversations with especially able people. Ilminster: Purple Field Press.

World Health Organisation (WHO) (1948) Preamble to the Constitution of the World Health Organization as adopted by the International Health Conference, New York, 19–22 June 1946; signed on 22 July 1946 by the representatives of 61 States (Official Records of the World Health Organization, no. 2, p. 100) and entered into force on 7 April 1948.

CHAPTER 5

Occupation and long-term neurological conditions

5.1 Introduction

Occupation is the foundation of occupational therapy, yet this relatively straightforward assertion becomes inordinately complex in practice. Challenges exist for occupational therapists in the application of the theoretical concepts of occupation to the accurate identification of occupational needs and the development of person-centred and meaningful occupational goals. Within this chapter occupation is considered within the constructs of doing, being, becoming and belonging and in the context of unpredictable and life-changing progressive neurological disease. Personal narratives are used throughout the chapter to illustrate the broader context of occupation in practice.

5.2 Defining occupation

Theoretical models of occupational therapy define occupation within three domains of self-care, productivity and leisure (Law et al., 1997, p. 34). Within this theoretical framework the focus is predominantly on the 'doing' aspects of the tasks which people carry out within their everyday lives. The main emphasis is placed on the execution of the task with secondary consideration of elements of performance capacity which may inhibit or restrict successful completion of the particular activity. This approach however provides little understanding of the meaning or purpose that engagement in such tasks brings to the person (Preston, 2009).

Throughout this book occupation will be considered within Wilcock's (1999) model of occupations for doing, being, becoming and belonging. Aspects of personal effectiveness, importance or worth attached to the task and the amount of enjoyment or satisfaction gained from participation all contribute to the level of motivation and willingness for a person to engage in activity (Preston et al., 2014).

Occupational Therapy and Neurological Conditions, First Edition. Edited by Jenny Preston and Judi Edmans.
© 2016 John Wiley & Sons, Ltd. Published 2016 by John Wiley & Sons, Ltd.

Diagnosis with a long-term neurological condition can significantly impact on the choice and potential abilities to engage in occupations which people find meaningful as can be seen within the following example (Preston, 2009):

> Maureen:
> So, it, it's, I mean it's [MS] played a big role in my life. What I've done and what I've not done, I mean I've never been abroad, I've only been down in England, three times…and…I don't make plans. Even when the children were small I never made plans to go anywhere, because I knew that every day that there would be something going on with me. I remember when eh, we had made a plan to rent a car and go away…and…I got neuralgia in my face. It's just, the pain, and I couldn't go anywhere. I remember going to eh, Arran, and the pain in my legs with just sitting in the car…and…I mean I wasn't doing anything…and we went out for a little walk round about to see what was going on…and eh, I was in agony, but the children were small, and I had to do it for the children. (Preston, 2009)

5.3 Occupational patterns

Occupational patterns develop over time and within certain socio-cultural norms of how the specific occupation is to be performed (Erlandsson and Christiansen, 2015). Analysis of occupational patterns therefore requires the occupational therapist to consider the past occupations as well as the future occupations of the person living with a long-term neurological condition (Erlandsson and Christiansen, 2015). Occupations will change and be adapted as people transition through life stages, and the meanings attributed will continue to evolve (Erlandsson and Christiansen, 2015).

People living with a long-term neurological condition may reflect on their previous occupations prior to the diagnosis often ascribing occupational change to the impairments and associated limitations of subsequent disease progression. Fraser provides an illustration of how his occupations have changed over time, and what this means for him, further to a diagnosis of multiple sclerosis (MS):

> Well…I was like working since I was a wee boy, you know like when I was 9 years old I worked for a milk run until I was 12, then when I was 12 I worked on the farms so, I was always used to going about all the time, hardly in the house, eh…, I just liked to be the one that provided for my family, when I couldn't do that, that kind of got to me… (Preston, 2009)

For others like Maureen, reflection on her current occupations helps her to understand her previous limitations within the context of her difficulties as a young woman prior to a diagnosis of MS:

> But now, now that I think about it, eh, what was going on with me, I mean I thought a lot of the time I was stupid and was slow. Um…but I wasn't stupid, and I know that. You just, now I can start putting things in place…that, this is happening to me because of the thingmy [MS]…um, so…I mean I've been able to sort of put things into place, where if you had had this interview with me when I was in my teens, I would have had a different eh opinion of what was going on with me and eh…I knew, I knew that I couldn't work. I wasn't…, nobody could depend on me. (Preston et al., 2014)

The nature of occupational patterns may develop a certain regularity, predictability, or consistency determined by the person living with a long-term neurological condition, for example changing bed linen every Monday, weekly shopping, or going to the hairdresser once a month (Erlandsson and Christiansen, 2015, p. 125). Society and culture may also influence these predictable patterns or routines such as going to church on Sundays. Routines are defined as 'occupations with established sequences and provide an orderly structure for daily living' (Erlandsson and Christiansen, 2015, p. 123).

Habits and routines are woven into the fabric of our personal and social lives as humans, and it is hard to get through the day without encountering some element of habitual behaviour (Graybiel, 2008). Habits are largely learned from repeated behaviours over the course of a period of days or years until they become fixed (Graybiel, 2008). The relationship between habit and long-term neurological conditions is not yet fully understood and as well as the implications for occupational therapy practice. However helpful as habits can be in daily life, they can become dominant and intrusive in neurological conditions such as Huntington's disease (HD) or exaggerated in some forms of Parkinson's (Graybiel, 2008).

Occupational patterns support people living with a long-term neurological condition to (Matuska and Christiansen, 2008):

- Meet basic needs and which are necessary for personal health and safety
- Have rewarding and self-affirming relationships with others
- Feel engaged, challenged and competent
- Create meaning and a satisfactory personal identity
- Organise time and energy to meet important personal goals and personal renewal.

Occupational balance occurs when there is equal participation in physical, cognitive, social and rest occupations (although the actual amount of time spent in each can be different) and when the individual finds meaning and value within the occupations in which they engage (Håkansson et al., 2006). Occupational balance is a dynamic process which requires a combination of occupations which are self-chosen and those which are required in response to daily habits and routine, or those expected from others (Håkansson et al., 2006). In order for an individual to achieve occupational balance, the person must perceive that they have the necessary competence and control to allow them to engage in personally meaningful occupations (Håkansson et al., 2006).

5.4 Doing, being, becoming and belonging

Occupation is the synthesis of doing, being and becoming that is central to everyday life and is necessary for adaptation and survival (Creek, 2003, p. 32). Wilcock's (1999) model provides a structure for the occupational therapist to explore and understand a person's unique relationship between an individual task/activity (doing) with their sense of self (being), ability to realise future aspirations (becoming) and a sense of inclusion in society (belonging).

5.4.1 Occupations for doing

> Doing is the medium through which people engage in occupations, and the skills and abilities needed for doing accumulate over time. Doing involves engaging in occupations that are personally meaningful but not necessarily purposeful, healthy or organised. Doing involves being actively engaged, either overtly (i.e. observable, physical) or tacitly (i.e. mental or spiritual). Doing follows broadly similar patterns across the population, and humans are able to adapt their doing to greater and lesser degrees according to circumstance. (Hitch et al., 2014)

Doing is an essential part of being human as 'people spend their lives almost constantly engaged in purposeful "doing" even when free of obligation or necessity' (Wilcock, 1999). When considering 'doing' it is important to identify the broad range of activities a person may engage in and the meaning and importance they attribute to these activities/tasks is fully explored and understood. Living with a long-term neurological condition can impact on all aspects of the person's ability to 'do' and in turn their sense of being, becoming and belonging.

Graeme offers some insight into what it meant for him when his walking ability changed due to MS. Graeme illustrates meaning through his comparison to child development when he was unable to perform what he believed to be a simple everyday function:

> I think because sometimes I can't do basic things like walk, you know, that takes all the confidence away from you that eh, I'll say to myself, you know it sounds stupid but kids at 3 year old, 4 year old walk about, and I'm blooming struggling to walk you know, I have got an illness but why the hell should I not be able to do that? (Preston, 2009)

For Grace, her continued engagement despite her difficulties with balance reflects her motivation to master aspects of doing within her routines:

> And that's, that's what I do, like um...I've seen a simple, well maybe it's not so simple like putting the curtains up, but I always think to myself how am I going to do that or see even painting, I'll say to myself right how am I going to paint that skirting board or whatever else, and I can't bend down because then I would fall over you see, so if you sit long enough I think I could get a chair and I could paint the skirting board sitting on a chair. With these kinds of problems I can always sort of find an answer. (Preston, 2009)

Capacity for doing relies on aspects of physical, cognitive and affective skills to allow the person living with a long-term neurological condition to carry out the actions, and monitor and modify the process as necessary (Hocking, 2011). Attitudes and beliefs shape the way things are done and how the knowledge and skills are applied to the occupation. Capacities change over time and can be acquired, maintained or honed through engagement in occupation (Hocking, 2011). Changes can also occur in knowledge, skills and attitudes in response to progressive neurological conditions.

5.4.2 Occupations for being

> Being is the sense of who someone is as an occupational and human being. It encompasses the meanings they invest in life, and their unique physical, mental, and social capacities and abilities. Occupation may provide a focus for being, but it also exists independently of it during reflection and self-discovery. Being is expressed through consciousness, creativity and the roles people assume in life. Ideally, individuals are able to exercise agency and choice in their expression of being, but this is not always possible or even desirable. (Hitch et al., 2014)

Below Diana describes her relationship with her friends and her need for them to see her as who she really is, independent of her diagnosis with MS:

> Probably because I don't want them feeling sorry for me. ...Yeah I don't want them feeling sorry for me, I want them to be my friends because they want to be my friend, not because oh I've got to go round and help Diana with this or help Diana with that. I'm not that type of person. Not that type of person. I prefer to do something in return. If somebody does something for me, I do something for them. I know that maybe sounds wrong, but that's me, that's me. ...that's who I am, who I am. (Preston et al., 2014)

Within the construct of 'being' the emphasis is on the experience of the occupation and the feelings it brings to the person living with a long-term neurological condition (Hammell, 2004). Being contributes to the development of occupational identity and the roles that people living with a long-term neurological condition inhabit within their everyday lives which in turn shapes the occupations in which people engage (Kielhofner, 2002, p. 73). As capacity changes for people living with a long-term neurological condition this may impact on their choice of occupations and their sense of occupational identity. Capacity in the sense of being relates to the 'innate and perhaps underdeveloped potential, aptitude, ability, talent, trait, or power with which each individual is endowed' (Wilcock, 2006).

At first glance, Maureen seems to describe her despair at not being able to cook for her family:

> And, um...I always cooked for my children and my husband. I never used tins. I used one tin a week, of food, and that was baked beans! Because I always cooked for my children and my husband, produced good food for myself. In the end up, before I was actually diagnosed with MS...I couldn't peel a potato, and I broke my heart. And then, it sounds silly not being able to peel a potato, I...(laugh) I sat and I cried myself silly that I couldn't peel a potato. (Preston, 2009)

However when the occupational therapist suggested that Maureen could use ready-prepared vegetables from the supermarket, it became apparent that Maureen's distress was due to her perception of being unable to fulfil her role as a mother, who, according to her own beliefs, had a duty to provide wholesome food for her family. By focussing on the practical aspects of food preparation alone the occupational therapist was unable to capture the subsequent meanings associated with this task for Maureen.

An important aspect of being, particularly for people living with degenerative neurological disease is the sense of 'being as existing' and the need for time and space as a means of self-discovery, thinking and reflection, or time to just 'be' (Hitch et al., 2014). People living with long-term neurological conditions need time to sit with their emotions, and take a break from life to reconfigure their individual sense of being as a pre-requisite for further active engagement (Hitch et al., 2014). Maureen offers an example of her personal reflections:

MAUREEN: I think, I think, eh, I'm not quite as 'me'.
RESEARCHER: Tell me more about that.
MAUREEN: Me, being the self-conscious, of what is going on, or me being um…as judging myself, I judge myself an awful lot, I know that, you know, um, but…I'm getting better at saying 'it doesn't matter'. (Preston, 2009)

Being rests on consciousness and creativity, and it is this subjective experience of consciousness or recognition of the self which is essential for engagement in occupational behaviour (Wilcock, 2006). People living with long-term neurological conditions may need to be supported to find new ways of doing things which allow them to create meaningful and satisfying lives (Preston et al., 2014). This however relies on the development of skills in planning, task prioritisation and problem solving, all of which may become compromised with long-term neurological conditions (Preston et al., 2014).

5.4.3 Occupations for becoming

> Becoming is the perpetual process of growth, development, and change that reside within a person throughout their life. It is directed by goals and aspirations which can arise through choice or necessity, from the individual or from groups. Regular modifications and revisions of goals and aspirations help to maintain momentum in becoming, as does the opportunity to experience new or novel situations and challenges. (Hitch et al., 2014)

Becoming is the dimension related to change and development, incorporating changes in relationships over time and throughout a person's lifetime (Wilcock, 2006). Becoming is a process with cycles of achieving goals and aspirations before setting new ones (Hitch et al., 2014). Hammell (2004) describes becoming as the process of people 'envisioning future selves and possible lives'. For Audrey her future hopes lie in the search for a cure for MS as she embarks on a clinical drug trial:

> I have tried various 'cures' unsuccessfully obviously, but I will try anything…I'm about to set sail on the cannabis trail, I hope, um, that is a trial I am aware of that, but if it is successful then it is a trail I shall be on. I have found it very frustrating to hear of people having cures, there's one in Oxford, one somewhere else, I can't quite remember where, um, and these were trials for a cure, there isn't one, at all, and no one is going to put me off, even at my age, trying, to, at least have a better…um,…state of living. I am a very independent person. (Preston, 2009)

However becoming does not always bring about improvement and the gap between a person's goals and actual achievements can be painfully evident

(Hitch et al., 2014). For Jennifer, it seemed that her dream of becoming a wife would no longer be fulfilled as her partner could not cope with the diagnosis of MS:

> I felt that I'm a wee bit, I've always been choosy, eh I've only ever really liked one person since I was a wee girl (laughs) and that's kinda, cause he doesn't seem to be able to deal with this [MS], I was going out with him when I found out I had this and he just kinda seemed to deal with it by just drinking too much and things have happened, he's moved away to the other end of the town, I haven't seen him for about 6 months, eh, I don't think we'll find our way back after this but you know, he just can't seem to deal with it…I don't really want to go out with anybody else. (Preston, 2009)

Living with a long-term neurological condition may require an acceptance that life has changed, with discontinuity of the former self and occupations and reconstruction of a new self. This may not necessarily mean a better self with evidence that for some people living with a long-term neurological condition this emerges as an unwanted self (Preston et al., 2014). This example is provided by Richard who reflects on his life after 40 years of living with MS:

> …certainly my ego has taken a knock over the years…um…yeah it has um…you're not…I'm not the man I used to be, that's how I feel. (Preston, 2009)

5.4.4 Occupations for belonging

> Belonging is a sense of connectedness to other people, places, cultures, communities, and times. It is the context within which occupations occur, and a person may experience multiple belongings at the same time. Relationships are essential to belonging, whether they be with a person, place, group, or other factor. A sense of reciprocity, mutuality, and sharing characterise belonging relationships, whether they are positive or negative. (Hitch et al., 2014)

Avril offers some insight into her sense of belonging within the MS community:

> People say 'how can you keep just going to MS?' I say well the thing is I was 23 when I took MS, I'm 58 now. I've had it 35 years so I've had it longer than I have had just living without it. So I say that is part of my life that I have it. (Preston et al., 2014)

While Richard has continued to value his relationships with his former colleagues, he has come to realise that aspects of connectedness and reciprocity no longer exist as he becomes more aware of the changing context after he left work:

> I even meet my colleagues sometimes, my ex-colleagues but I've got nothing in common with them, the only thing we had was the job, but that (laughs)…socially you don't want to do that, discuss the job, people that you've known for years…and that's all you've got in common, they've got their own problems, families and all the rest of it and it becomes more and more difficult to…um…talk to people…yeah…. (Preston, 2009)

Graeme also felt a lack of connectedness with his friends since his diagnosis with MS:

> Eh, I have lost friends since I had MS eh, but basically…they weren't friends, you know, they just sort of never came, I think they were so embarrassed about it. I don't know why.

Researcher: What do you think they were embarrassed of?

I don't know, I don't know, well maybe because I was eh in a wheelchair at one time, eh like all the time and eh I think that puts a lot of people say well, I'm walking about with a guy in a wheelchair, it's eh...embarrassing you know, but, I don't think it's embarrassing because I'm in a wheelchair eh, you know. (Preston, 2009)

5.5 Occupational dysfunction

Occupational dysfunction describes the problems people may have with performing occupations (Reed, 2015). Kielhofner (1995) stated that 'we recognise occupational dysfunction when an individual has difficulty performing, organising, or choosing occupations'. Whiteford (2000) conceptualises occupational dysfunction 'either as a by-product of non-resolved occupational disruption, as a result of specific occupational performance deficits, or as arising from a prolonged state of occupational deprivation'. Occupational dysfunction 'is a phenomenon that is nested in a complex of factors all of which reflect and contribute to sustaining the performance, patterns of behaviour, identities, choices and so on, that reflect a life in trouble' (Kielhofner, 1995, p. 156). Occupational dysfunction occurs at different levels within the International Classification of Function (ICF) framework (World Health Organisation [WHO], 2002) as illustrated in Table 5.1.

Occupational justice is an umbrella term which describes a range of restrictions to participation in occupation (Townsend and Wilcock, 2004). Occupational justice is developed from an understanding that 'people want to do, need to do, and can do considering their personal and social circumstances' (Stadnyk et al., 2010). According to Wilcock and Townsend (2009, p. 330) 'an occupationally just world is envisaged as one that would be governed in a way that enables individuals to flourish by doing what they decide is most meaningful and useful to themselves and their families, communities and nations'.

Occupational apartheid occurs 'where opportunities for occupation are afforded to some individuals and restricted to others based on personal characteristics such as race, disability, gender, age, nationality, religion, social status, sexuality and so on' (Kronenberg and Pollard, 2005).

Occupational disruption is the term used to describe a state 'in which occupational engagement is temporarily disturbed due to significant life events, environmental changes, becoming ill or sustaining an injury from which full recovery is expected' (Whiteford, 2000). Given the temporary nature of occupational disruption and with supportive conditions, it usually resolves by itself (Whiteford, 2000).

Occupational deprivation describes a 'state of preclusion from engagement in occupations of necessity and/or meaning due to factors that stand outside the immediate control of the individual' (Whiteford, 2000). Occupational deprivation can have a long-term effect on the individual's overall health and well-being.

Table 5.1 Examples of occupational dysfunction applied to the ICF levels of disability.

Health condition	Impairment	Activity	Participation
George was diagnosed with Parkinson's.	He now experiences a marked tremor in his left hand.	Due to the tremor, George finds it difficult to cut and eat his food. His wife helps on occasions at home to allow him to eat while his food is hot.	George previously enjoyed participating in family gatherings and social events which involved eating out in restaurants. George is embarrassed about his tremor and feels that everybody is looking at his hand shaking. He is afraid that he will not be able to cut up his food and eat it without making a mess. George now chooses not to go out for meals with his family and friends.
Sarah was diagnosed with MND.	Due to the weakening of her neck muscles, Sarah is finding it hard to hold her head up	Sarah had been enjoying going out in the car with her husband. However because of the difficulties with her head control, she finds that now she can only sit in the car for very short journeys.	Sarah enjoyed visiting local beauty spots and the freedom of 'getting away from the door'. Sarah would look forward to spontaneously bumping into people and chatting. Sarah now spends most of her time within her own home. Her social interaction with others is now generally planned and with a much smaller circle of family and friends. Sarah now goes out in the car for essential trips such as medical appointments.
John was diagnosed with HD	He is aware that at times he finds it hard to make decisions.	John works in the financial industry and has the responsibility of managing 15 staff and a £2 million budget.	John was very concerned that his difficulties making decisions might impact on his work and his company. John did not want to be responsible for making the wrong decisions and decided to give up work.
Sandra was diagnosed with MS.	Sandra experiences difficulties with urinary frequency and urinary urgency.	Sandra used to enjoy shopping trips with her friends.	Sandra likes to plan her shopping trips around the location of toileting facilities to give her the confidence to know that she can access the toilet quickly. This means that she tends to restrict herself to familiar shopping facilities and opts not to join her friends when they visit unfamiliar venues.

Source: Adapted from: WHO, 2002, p. 17.

Occupational marginalisation refers to the 'exclusion from participation in occupations based on "invisible" norms and expectations about who should participate in what occupations, how, when, and why' (Durocher et al., 2014). Occupational marginalisation is further described as 'situations where individuals or groups may not be afforded choice to participate in valid occupations, and may be relegated to those that are less prestigious or allow little choice or control' (Stadnyk et al., 2010) or little opportunity for decision-making (Townsend and Wilcock, 2004).

Consider the following situations encountered within neurological practice and how they impact on aspects of occupational performance, occupational dysfunction and occupational justice:

- Fraser is no longer able to engage in paid employment as a consequence of his neurological condition. He reflects on the experience of attending for an assessment for Incapacity Benefit:

  > ...and I hate like being on benefits...because I just like providing for my family and that, I never wanted benefits, and then when I did eventually claim...I got on Incapacity Benefit. There was a fella interviewing me and my wife was with me...and huh, I did really feel like just pulling him over his desk and hitting him one...so I said to him 'don't sit there and look down your nose at me', I said, 'I've worked all my days' that really got to me. (Preston, 2009)

- Julia and her husband enjoy cruising for their annual holiday as they feel that it is an appropriate option for Julia due to her reduced mobility as a consequence of HD. They particularly enjoy the excursions and experiencing different cities and cultures. On a recent trip, Julia found that when she attempted to leave the ship to visit one of the ports there were difficulties securing the bridge which allowed her to disembark the ship while using her wheelchair. The proposed solution offered by the ship's personnel was that Julia would be lifted off the ship in her wheelchair by four members of the crew. Julia was 'horrified' at the thought of this and opted to accept a 'piggy back' from her husband instead. Julia felt quite humiliated by this as the other passengers looked on, and she decided that she would not participate in any further excursions ashore during this trip.

- For Jennifer the practical problems associated with her neurological condition seemed insurmountable as she described why she was unable to meet her friend as often as she would like. Environmental barriers contributed to Jennifer's worries about how she would manage to get to the toilet in her friend's home:

  > ...which is another reason I don't want to go up to my friends for a drink, even in her house because she's got stairs but she's got no banister, she's got nothing to hold on to, my balance, and it's quite embarrassing and she's 'oh just say to [friend's husband]' and I say 'I'm not wanting to ask your husband every time I need to go up to the bathroom, you know to hold on to your arm or something, it's embarrassing...'. (Preston, 2009)

- Eric was diagnosed with motor neurone disease (MND) and his wife is no longer able to support him at home. Eric moved into a care home as he was concerned that his continually changing needs would impact on his wife's overall health and well-being. Eric previously enjoyed painting and found that this allowed him some opportunity for creativity and relief from the stresses of his demanding career. Eric has continued to paint despite the deterioration apparent in his medical condition. When Eric moved into the care home, he was advised that there was insufficient storage for his easel and his art materials could not be accommodated within the care home due to the 'enhanced fire risk'.
- Derek has a diagnosis of Parkinson's. Recently he tripped at home and broke his arm. Derek is experiencing a temporary disruption to his daily activities, that is dressing, cooking and eating due to the application of a plaster to support healing. Derek is keen to have the plaster removed so that he can resume his normal activities.

5.6 Occupational adaptation

The personal narratives used throughout this chapter have illustrated how occupational identity and occupational competence are developed and realised in response to diagnosis with a long-term neurological condition (Kielhofner, 2008). Occupational adaptation is defined as the extent to which a person's perceived identity corresponds to his or her competence performing occupations of personal importance in a relevant environment (Lexell et al., 2011). It is an ongoing process where a person's experiences of his or her previous occupational adaptations will influence novel challenges encountered in the future, and thereby influence his or her ongoing engagement in occupations (Lexell et al., 2011).

People living with long-term neurological conditions are forced to repeat their adaptations due to disease-induced deterioration (Lexell et al., 2011). It is important that the occupational therapist understands this process of adaptation when considering meaningful occupational therapy interventions (Lexell et al., 2011). Patterns of occupational adaptation are apparent for people living with long-term neurological conditions which can be classified within three key categories of adapting occupations to preserve the former sense of self, adapting occupations to find the new sense of self and adapting occupations to live with the changed sense of self (Lexell et al., 2011).

Some distinct behaviours may be associated with adaptive responses as adapted from Lexell et al. (2011):

Adapting occupations to preserve the former sense of self:

- Concealing shortcomings by explaining away difficulties in performance, for example I always trip over that step, it must be my shoes.
- Challenging their ability to perform different tasks with the aim of preserving the capable self, for example taking on a more demanding job role despite being exhausted at the end of the work day.

- Making temporary adaptations to their occupations, for example I'll ask my husband to help with making dinner just for the next few weeks until I get back on my feet.
- Changing the means of performing an occupation that enabled them to stay engaged in those that they prioritised, for example I have a shower in the afternoon now because I am too tired in the morning by the time I get the kids ready for school.
- Refusing to take on the identity of a person with a disability, for example there's no way I'm using a wheelchair, I don't want to look disabled.
  Adapting occupations to find the new sense of self:
- Seeking occupations that support feelings of capability, for example I've always been good at painting.
- Re-engaging in former activities which they had discontinued, for example it's years since I have been to yoga, I'd forgotten how much I enjoy it.
- Identifying new occupations which contribute to feelings of capability and success, for example I really wasn't very sure about joining the gym, but I'm amazed how much more energy I have once I have been.
- Avoiding occupations that may result in failure, for example I have burned myself so many times now that I just don't do the ironing any more. Thank goodness for that ironing service!
- Avoiding occupations or turn down occupations in which they used to be involved but were no longer able to be certain they could control, for example I don't go out with my friends now as I don't know how much walking will be involved and I'm scared I can't keep up with them.
- Avoiding receiving assistance and striving for independence in occupations for as long as possible, for example my mother-in-law has offered to pick the kids up from school, but I want to be able to do that by myself for as long as I can.
- Allowing other people to influence their choice of occupational adaptations, for example the occupational therapist suggested I get a seat for the shower to reduce the risk of losing my balance when I am washing my hair.
- Striving to avoid stigma.
  Adapting occupations to live with the changed sense of self:
- Planning and preparation for occupations, for example only visiting familiar places and people who make them feel secure.
- Keeping to familiar routines, for example grocery shopping.
- Ignoring shortcomings in their own performance and focussing on the possibilities they have in the future, for example maybe I don't clean the bathroom as often as I should at the moment but once I move to a new house and I don't have to climb stairs that will all change.
- Reluctance to use their energy bothering about occupations they could no longer perform or engage in, for example cutting the grass is my husband's job, I've got far more important things to do in the garden.
- Focussing on occupations that supported the sense of self, providing a sense of well-being, for example I know I will be exhausted after going away for the weekend, but it's worth it just to relax on the beach.

- Becoming advocates or representatives for other people with disability.
- Accepting help as a process of adaptation, for example now that I am used to the wheelchair I can join in with the family again when we go out for the day.

5.7 Defining occupational goals

A fundamental component of occupational therapy philosophy and practice involves recognition of the importance of an individual's meaningful daily-life experiences. As occupational therapists we are interested in facilitating the development of skills and abilities which allow people living with a long-term neurological condition to achieve or return to activities which are personally meaningful (Eschenfelder, 2005). The issue is how therapists come to recognise activities and experiences which are meaningful to people living with long-term neurological conditions and how we go about incorporating this understanding in our practice (Eschenfelder, 2005). Therapists have traditionally developed goals that focus on impairments such as improving balance or range of movement (Randall and McEwen, 2000). Goal setting during occupational therapy intervention may be enhanced by exploring the client's meaningful life experiences including past and current roles, responsibilities and activities which are particularly meaningful to individual client's their families or caregivers (Eschenfelder, 2005).

People are likely to make the greatest gains when therapy and the related goals focus on activities that are meaningful to them and that will make a difference in their lives (Randall and McEwen, 2000). Occupational therapists need to consider how meaningful life experience may help in the development of treatment goals that are more meaningful to the individual client (Eschenfelder, 2005).

The process of defining meaningful, achievable goals should be a collaborative one between the person living with the long-term neurological condition, possibly their family/carer and the occupational therapist (Randall and McEwen, 2000). For goals to be truly person-centred, they should be relevant to the person's desired outcomes, not to what the therapist thinks is 'best' for the client (Randall and McEwen, 2000). Dunn (1993) encouraged occupational therapists to develop a new perspective about the meaning and usefulness of independence. Rather than asking whether a person is independent in tasks, perhaps we need to ask what conditions are necessary to enable the person to accomplish the task. In this perspective we assume that the person is capable and consider what factors in the environment might be needed to support task or performance (Dunn, 1993).

In practice, therapists are involved with people living with long-term neurological conditions who are experiencing significant loss or changes in function and who are facing meaning-related issues (Eschenfelder, 2005). Life roles and domains, activities, relationships and experience are important areas for discovering individual meanings for people living with long-term neurological conditions

(Eschenfelder, 2005). The growing use of narratives allows therapists to explore these meanings in a clinical setting. Therapists can begin to ask the person and their family what they need and want to do in their lives (Dunn, 1993). They can investigate what is important, desirable or pleasurable for the person and then accept and use this information when planning interventions (Dunn, 1993).

5.8 Self-evaluation questions

1 What are the three domains of occupation described within the theoretical models of occupational therapy?
2 How does diagnosis with a long-term neurological condition impact on the choice and potential abilities to engage in meaningful occupations?
3 How do occupational patterns develop?
4 How do occupational patterns support occupational performance?
5 How can habit contribute to occupational dysfunction in neurological conditions?
6 What are the four constructs within Wilcock's (1999) model?
7 How do we recognise occupational dysfunction in people living with long-term neurological conditions?
8 What is occupational adaptation?
9 How can occupational therapists contribute to the development of meaningful occupational goals?
10 When does occupational balance occur?

References

Creek J (2003) Occupational therapy defined as a complex intervention. London: College of Occupational Therapists.

Dunn W (1993) Measurement of function: actions for the future. The American Journal of Occupational Therapy, 47(4):357–359.

Durocher E, Gibson BE and Rappolt S (2014) Occupational justice: a conceptual review. Journal of Occupational Science, 21(4):418–430.

Erlandsson LK and Christiansen C (2015) The complexity and patterns of human occupations. In Christiansen C, Baum C and Bass J (Eds) Occupational therapy: performance, participation and well-being, 4th Edition. Thorofare, NJ: Slack Incorporated, pp. 113–127.

Eschenfelder V (2005) Shaping the goal setting process in OT: the role of meaningful occupation. Physical and Occupational Therapy in Geriatrics, 23(4):67–81.

Graybiel A (2008) Habits, rituals and the evaluative brain. The Annual Review of Neuroscience, 31:359–387.

Håkansson C, Dahlinivanoff S and Sonn U (2006) Achieving balance in everyday life. Journal of Occupational Science, 13(1):74–82.

Hammell KW (2004) Dimensions of meaning in the occupations of daily life. Canadian Journal of Occupational Therapy, 71:296–305.

Hitch D, Pépin G and Stagnitti K (2014) In the footsteps of Wilcock, part one: the evolution of doing, being, becoming, and belonging. Occupational Therapy in Health Care, 28(3):231–246.

Hocking C (2011) The challenge of occupation: describing the things people do. Journal of Occupational Science, 16(3):140–150.

Kielhofner G (1995) A model of human occupation: therapy and application, 2nd Edition. Baltimore, MD: Lippincott Williams & Wilkins.

Kielhofner G (2002) Habituation: patterns of daily occupation. In Kielhofner G (Ed.) Model of human occupation theory and application, 3rd Edition. Baltimore, MD: Lippincott Williams & Wilcott, pp. 63–80.

Kielhofner G (2008) Model of Human Occupation: theory and application, 4th Edition. Baltimore, MD: Lippincott, Williams & Wilkins.

Kronenberg F and Pollard N (2005) Overcoming occupational apartheid: a preliminary exploration of the political nature of occupational therapy. In Kronenberg F, Algado SS and Pollard N (Eds) Occupational therapy without borders: learning from the spirit of survivors. Toronto, ON: Elsevier Churchill Livingstone, pp. 58–86.

Law M, Polatajko H, Baptiste S and Townsend E (1997) Core concepts of occupational therapy. Enabling occupation: an occupational therapy perspective. Ottawa, ON: Canadian Association of Occupational Therapists, pp. 29–56.

Lexell E, Iwarsson S and Lund M (2011) Occupational adaptation in people with multiple sclerosis. OTJR: Occupation, Participation and Health, 31(3):127–134.

Matuska KM and Christiansen CH (2008) A proposed model of lifestyle balance. Journal of Occupational Science, 15(1):9–19.

Preston JA (2009) Executive function and multiple sclerosis: implications for occupational therapy practice. PhD Thesis, Glasgow Caledonian University.

Preston J, Ballinger C and Gallagher H (2014) Understanding the lived experience of people with multiple sclerosis and dysexecutive syndrome. British Journal of Occupational Therapy, 77(10):484–490.

Randall K and McEwen I (2000) Writing patient-centred functional goals. Physical Therapy, 80(12):1197–1203.

Reed KL (2015) Key occupational therapy concepts in the Person-Occupational-Environment-Performance model: their origin and historical use in the occupational therapy literature. In Christiansen C, Baum C and Bass J (Eds) Occupational therapy: performance, participation and well-being, 4th Edition. Thorofare, NJ: Slack Incorporated, pp. 565–648.

Stadnyk R, Townsend E and Wilcok A (2010) Occupational justice. In Christiansen CH and Townsend EA (Eds) Introduction to occupation: the art and science of living, 2nd Edition. Upper Saddle River, NJ: Pearson Education, pp. 329–358.

Townsend E and Wilcock A (2004) Occupational justice and client-centred practice: a dialogue in progress. Canadian Journal of Occupational Therapy, 71(2):75–87.

Whiteford G (2000) Occupational deprivation: global challenge in the new millennium. British Journal of Occupational Therapy, 63(5):200–204.

Wilcock AA (1999) Reflections on doing, being and becoming… Australian Occupational Therapy Journal, 46(1):1–11.

Wilcock A (2006) An occupational perspective of health, 2nd Edition. Thorofare, NJ: SLACK Incorporated.

Wilcock A and Townsend E (2009) Occupational justice. In Crepeau EB, Cohn ES and Schell BAB (Eds) Willard and Spackman's occupational therapy, 11th Edition. Philadelphia, PA: Lippincott Williams & Wilkins, pp. 192–199.

World Health Organisation [WHO] (2002) Towards a common language for functioning, disability and health: ICF. Geneva: World Health Organisation.

CHAPTER 6

Identifying occupational performance enablers and deficits

6.1 Introduction

Occupational therapists are increasingly required to demonstrate the effectiveness of their interventions and articulate how their intervention adds value to the client journey and client experience. Despite an increasing selection of robust outcome measures it remains challenging for the occupational therapist, eager to evaluate the impact of their interventions, to know where to begin when considering outcome measurement in neurological rehabilitation. In this chapter we explore the need for measurement, the fundamentals of good measurement practice and review some key measurement tools, which contribute to the identification of occupational performance enablers and deficits for people living with a long-term neurological condition.

6.2 What is measurement?

Measurement is defined by Fawcett (2013) as follows: 'Measurement is the data obtained by measuring. Measuring is undertaken by therapists to ascertain the dimension (size), quantity (amount) or capacity of a trait, attribute or characteristic of a person that is required by the therapist to develop an accurate picture of the person's needs and problems to form a baseline for therapeutic intervention and/or to provide a measure of outcome. A measurement is obtained by applying a standard scale to variables, thus translating direct observations or client/priority reports to a numerical scoring system'.

Occupational Therapy and Neurological Conditions, First Edition. Edited by Jenny Preston and Judi Edmans.
© 2016 John Wiley & Sons, Ltd. Published 2016 by John Wiley & Sons, Ltd.

6.3 What are occupational therapy outcomes?

Outcomes are the end result of an intervention or action, or lack of it, on an individual, or on a population group. They are the changes that occur that may be attributed, to some degree, to the intervention (or lack of it). (College of Occupational Therapists, 2012)

6.3.1 Why measure?

Outcome measurement can demonstrate the effectiveness of occupational therapy intervention for people living with a long-term neurological condition at an individual level or as part of a wider population group guiding further decision-making and/or intervention. The use of outcome measures, especially standardised measures, allows occupational therapists to build up and use a body of evidence for occupational therapy (College of Occupational Therapists, 2012).

An outcome measure is a tool to measure or quantify this change. An initial assessment provides the baseline against which a later measurement can be compared when considering the outcome for the person living with a long-term neurological condition (College of Occupational Therapists, 2012).

Figure 6.1 demonstrates the three factors involved in measuring in clinical practice.

6.3.2 How to measure

A 'standardised' outcome measure (as for standardised assessment tools) has a set, unchanging procedure that must be used when carried out, as well as a consistent system for scoring. This ensures minimal variation in the way it is carried out at different times and by different testers. The scoring system may also have been normatively standardised, meaning that the test has been used with a very large group of similar people, giving an average score or range of expected scores that the tester and the service user can use to

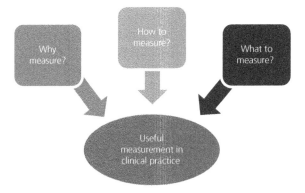

Figure 6.1 Understanding the three factors involved in measuring in clinical practice.

compare with their own results. Standardised tests have known levels of reliability, validity and utility, which ensure that therapists can select and use them appropriately and with confidence in the results. (College of Occupational Therapists, 2012)

6.3.3 What to measure

Examples of outcomes that can be measured include the following (College of Occupational Therapists, 2012):
- Improvements in health or quality of life (QOL)
- Improvements in function or level of independence
- Attainment of intervention goals
- Service user satisfaction
- Systems change such as reduced hospital length of stay, waiting lists and read-mission rates.

The occupational therapist will also be concerned with measuring outcomes for secondary purposes such as service management, service commissioning, information for central government, clinical audit and other research (College of Occupational Therapists, 2012; Figure 6.2).

6.4 Selecting the right measure

The quality of the measure relates to how well it has been constructed. A measure's construction, or its psychometric integrity, relates to the way in which the measure is designed and performs (British Society of Rehabilitation Medicine [BSRM], 2005; Table 6.1). This includes how the measure is standardised in the way it is used and if it has been validated to show change in a specific clinical population when compared to a normal population. The measure's reliability over time and between users also needs to have been objectively proven (Figure 6.3).

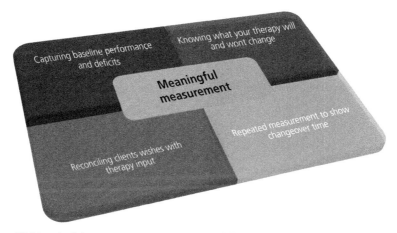

Figure 6.2 Meaningful measurement in occupational therapy practice.

Table 6.1 How to use measures in a meaningful way? Key questions and red flags.

	Key questions	Red flags
1. How 'good' is the measure?		
Is the measure reliable and valid?	• Does it give you the same outcome when used by different people (inter-rater reliability)? • Does it give you the same outcome when used by the same person at a different time (intra-rater reliability)? • Has the measure undergone a series of robust testing to prove it is a useful and valid tool within the clinical area intended? • Is it validated for use with your client population? • Is it meant to be used in a specific environment, in a particular way?	Read about how the measure has been formally evaluated. This is usually in the box or instruction book. If the measure is 'home grown' or has been developed within the department, it will usually not have been evaluated or proven to be reliable. This means that any results you get may not be meaningful or reproducible. *Don't use the measure:* • In a different way from the way it is designed, for example don't miss sections out, complete a team score on your own • If it is not validated for your client population, including age range and diagnosis • If it is intended to be used in a different environment as this will invalidate the results.
Does the measure have face validity?	• Does the measure capture what it is designed to measure? • Is it easy to understand? • Does the scoring method make sense? • Can you readily make sense of the results and what they mean?	Make sure you are choosing the right measure for the clinical question you want answering, for example if you want to know specifically about levels of fatigue, use a fatigue measure not a global ADL measure. *Don't use the measure:* • If you don't know how the results help you answer your clinical question • If you don't know how the results can help direct your interventions.
Is the measure sensitive enough?	• Is the measure sensitive to change over time? • Can it be used repeatedly or is there a test–retest learning effect? • Does the measure have a floor or ceiling effect where clients are either too impaired (floor) or perform too well (ceiling) for the measure to capture change? • Do changes on the measure indicate a clinically meaningful difference, that is what do the changes mean for the client? For example an increase of 5° range of movement may not make any difference to the person in their day-to-day tasks.	Some measures have more than one test version to avoid an improvement in the client score being a result of them learning the test! Use multiple versions as per the instructions As a rule, the more increments or points on a scale the measure has, the more sensitive it is. However, this also makes it more time consuming to score and more likely that you will need specific training to reliably differentiate between the increments on the scale When clients have both physical and cognitive impairments, 'clinically meaningful change' might prove different per person, for example a score of 20/20 on the Barthel ADL Index (Collin et al., 1988; Mahoney and Barthel, 1965) suggests the client is physically safe but might still require 24-hour care due to cognitive issues. You may wish to change the measurement you choose if the first time you use it the client is already very near the top or near the bottom.

2. Is the measure 'suitable' for you to use?

| Can the measure be used readily in your work place? | • Do you need space and kit to set up?
• How long does it take to use?
• Does it need to be scored by a team or one person?
• Do you need specific training to use it?
• How much does the measure and measurement kit cost?
• Do you need to be 'accredited' to use the measure? | It is now possible to watch the set-up and use of most measures in practice via media platforms such as YouTube. This is a very useful way to watch peers perform the test with clients, and flags up key aspects of space, kit and standardisation.

Some measures might be suitable for your client population but may prove prohibitive in relation to pre-use training commitments, for example AMPS (Fisher and Bray Jones, 2010a, 2010b) requires the scorer to undertake a 5-day training course and a period of case practice before the user is 'accredited' to use the measure.

Do not be tempted to use team scored measures as a sole clinician to save time. This will invalidate all results, meaning results can't be submitted to UK Rehabilitation Outcomes Collaborative (UK ROC, 2015) if required or shared across teams, for example UK FIM+FAM (Turner-Stokes et al., 1999b) must always be scored by the team who support the client over 24 hours. |
| Can the measure be easily communicated to others? | • Are your peers already using this measure?
• Can the results and outcomes from the measurement be readily conveyed and understood by others?
• Does the team think the effort of undertaking the measure is worth the added value it affords? | Being able to share measurement outcomes across teams allows changes in the client's performance to be accurately and readily communicated over time. This is particularly significant when a client's skills are declining as a sense of speed of deterioration will be objectively captured by a measure.

Remember that your clinical question might change over time, for example if the client's decline in performance is such that you need to refocus your intervention to support the family, then you need a measure to capture carer strain rather than the client's performance at that time. |

Source: Based on Turner-Stokes et al. (2012) and BSRM (2005).

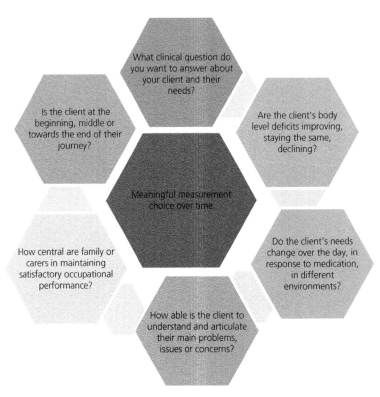

Figure 6.3 Client-centred decision-making: selecting the right measure at the right time.

6.5 Commonly used measures in neurological rehabilitation

The following section is intended to provide an overview of outcome measures commonly used by occupational therapists within neurological rehabilitation environments. The tools described are not exhaustive and intend to represent a contemporary range of measures that therapists may use or see in use at the time of publication.

All measures included have been evidenced as being reliable and valid in a neurologically impaired adult population. However, it is suggested that readers make use of all original references and up-to-date published work relating to the measure they wish to use in order that they understand the reach of its use. It is also prudent for therapists to appreciate that the world of measurement is dynamic and measures are continually being developed and evaluated for clinical use (Table 6.2).

6.5.1 Activities of daily living indices
The following three activities of daily living (ADL) indices have been grouped together due to their similarity (Table 6.3). Although not exclusively used by occupational therapists, all three ADL indices provide an easy snap-shop of performance across listed ADLs.

Table 6.2 Occupational therapy-specific outcome measures.

Assessment of Motor and Process Skills (AMPS) – activity-level measure

Brief overview *Domain measured,* *intended use, value* *of end result and* *suitable audience*	AMPS is an observational occupational therapy outcome measure designed to to evaluate an individual client's skills and deficits at an ***activity level***. The client is helped to choose two tasks that are undertaken in a familiar environment. Tasks are set up and carried out in a specified way, with no assistance provided by the observer unless unsafe task breakdown is seen. The outcome is a profile of occupational performance skills and deficits across personal and domestic activities of daily living (ADLs). AMPs outcomes can be shared with the client and commissioners to show client-level change. Results may also be readily transferred between AMPS raters, providing a reliable means of tracking occupational performance deficits across time and services.
Administration *For example, set-up* *and scoring,* *training* *requirements*	AMPS can be administered and scored in 1 hour or less and can be used in any relevant and familiar environment (clinical or community-based). Quality of performance is recorded on a 4-point scale across 16 motor and 20 process skills, providing a scale of motor and process ability compared to the norm. AMPS illustrates issues with performance such as increased physical effort, decreased efficiency, safety and risks taken offering predictive value regarding the need for physical assistance and supervision during ADLs. **AMPS can only be used by a registered occupational therapist**. To become a calibrated AMPS assessor, occupational therapists must undertake a 5-day course and complete a period of case examples. This creates a unique calibration profile for each scorer, and all results need to be added into a specific data system for results to be produced. AMPS assessors need to stay up to date and refresh if they have not used the measure for a number of years.
Key references	Fisher and Bray Jones (2010a, 2010b) and Fisher (1994, 1997)

Canadian Occupational Performance Measure (COPM) – activity and participation level measure

Brief overview *Domain measured,* *intended use, value* *of end result and* *suitable audience*	CPOM is a client centred measure which detects change in an individual client's reported self-perception of task performance and satisfaction with that performance over time. The COPM is administered using a face-to-face semi-structured interview that may include the caregiver if required. By validating areas of key concern and actively collaborating on therapy goals, COPM helps clients to remain focused and motivated to engage in therapy over time. Rescoring should be undertaken blind to avoid a placebo effect. Interview fatigue and misunderstanding of rating scales can influence reliability of numerical scores particularly with clients with some degree of cognitive impairment. Carers can help 'sense check' the process with clients with changeable insight or variable levels of performance. COPM outcomes can be shared with the client and commissioners to show the client's perceived change in performance and satisfaction with that performance over time.
Administration *For example, set-up* *and scoring,* *training* *requirements*	The COPM has a user manual that must be followed for scoring to be undertaken reliably. A COPM interview takes about 45 minutes to undertake and a five-step approach. A training DVD is also available. **Problem identification** A list of problems across self-care, productivity and leisure areas is recorded looking at what the client wants to do, needs to do or is expected to do **Problem weighting** All problems identified above are then scored on a 10-point visual analogue scale according to importance, with the top five problems identified and prioritised.

(continued)

Table 6.2 (Continued)

	Scoring Using a 10-point visual analogue scale the client then scores their perceived quality of performance and satisfaction with performance for the top five important problems. This generates a numerical value that can be used to benchmark the client's perceived performance over time. **Re-assessment and follow-up** Following a period of intervention, the COPM interview can be repeated to enable perceived change to be captured for the top five important problems and other problems to be reprioritised and scored as required. Follow-up includes a refresh of issues initially identified, agreement of self-help strategies and referral onto other team members as required.
Key references	Dedding et al. (2004) and Law et al. (1990, 2005)

Model of Human Occupation Screening Tool (MOHOST) – activity- and participation-level measure

Brief overview
Domain measured,
intended use, value
of end result and
suitable audience
	MOHOST aims to capture client-centred occupationally focused information, helping to inform an understanding of the client and their unique performance issues. The MOHOST is administered flexibly using a face-to-face semi-structured interview with self-reported performance where possible. This self-report is then reconciled via direct task observation and/or discussion with other caregivers. MOHOST is relevant to use within any speciality and is useful to capture occupational performance issues with clients who have limited ability to participate. Key areas that are captured represent the Model of Human Occupation (Kielhofner, 2002) dimensions of Volition, Habituation and Environment. MOHOST covers the following six sections:
	    1 Motivation for occupation
	    2 Pattern of occupation
	    3 Communication and interaction skills
	    4 Process skills
	    5 Motor skills
	    6 Environment
	with performance in each section captured by a further four sub sections that are scored using the FAIR systems. FAIR is a four-point standardised system used to describe circumstances of performance with one letter circled that best represents reported ability:
	    F = Facilitates occupational participation
	    A = Allows
	    I = Inhibits
	    R = Restricts
	Each subsection also has room for comments.
	Analysis of strengths and limitations are then summarised based on the profile found across all 24 subsections. MOHOST outcomes can be shared with the client and commissioners to show the client's change in performance over time.

Administration *For example, set-up* *and scoring,* *training* *requirements*	All MOHOST resources and user manuals are available on-line and must be followed to ensure objectivity of measurement. MOHOST workshops are also available but not a prerequisite to using the tool. A MOHOST interview and assessment may be conducted over a number of sessions and may include information from others sources as required.
Key references	Kielhofner (2002) and Parkinson et al. (2006)

Table 6.3 Commonly used activities of daily living indices.

Activities of Daily Living (ADL) Indices – activity- and participation-level measures including the following
- Barthel ADL Index
- Frenchay Activities Index
- Nottingham Extended ADL (NEADL) Index.

Brief overview	These three ADL Indices are client-centred measures that captures a client's
Domain measured,	self-reported task performance in a given task list over time.
intended use, value of	Using either a 3- or 4-point scale, the client chooses the number that best
end result and suitable	represents their participation in the given tasks.
audience	For example, NEADL Index:
	0 – Not at all
	1 – With help
	2 – Alone with difficulty
	3 – Alone easily
	Scores are then summed to provide a total score, the greater the score
	indicating a greater level of ability or participation in the ADL list.
	Outcomes are very easy for the client to understand and are popular
	measuring tools in busy clinical services.
Administration	Most of the aforementioned indices take about 5 minutes to complete and
For example, set-up	may be administered via a semi-structured interview, via observation or sent
and scoring, training	through the post and may include the caregiver if required.
requirements	If used over time, rescoring should be undertaken blind to avoid a placebo effect.
Key references	The Barthel ADL Index – Mahoney and Barthel (1965) and Wade and Collin (1988)
	Frenchay Activities Index – Holbrook and Skilbeck (1983)
	NEADL Index – Nouri and Lincoln (1987)

All three ADL indices have ecological validity and transferability and are able to be scored and rescored across services over time. Although there is no need for formal training to use each index, team members need to decide on the version of the index they are using plus understand and follow published guidelines for use. All three ADL indices are limited in relation to their sensitivity and do not take into consideration cognitive issues during physical performance.

The Functional Independence Measure and Functional Assessment Measure

The Functional Independence Measure (FIM) scale was developed to capture a deeper level of ADL performance due to both physical and cognitive disabilities, scoring the level of assistance required for an individual to perform ADL. The Functional Assessment Measure (FAM) was subsequently added to look at additional issues around cognition, communication and participation and both are frequently used by in-patient neuro-rehabilitation teams. The combined UK version of the FIM + FAM is a reportable output for the UKROC database (Table 6.4).

Table 6.4 Functional Independence Measure and Functional Assessment Measure.

UK FIM + FAM – activity- and participation-level measures

Brief overview *Domain measured,* *intended use, value* *of end result and* *suitable audience*	The FIM is an observer reported ADL scale. It includes 18 items, of which 13 items are physical domains based on the Barthel Index and 5 items are cognition items. Each item is scored from 1 to 7 based on the level of independence.

7	Complete independence	Fully independent
6	Modified independence	Requiring the use of a device but no physical help
5	Supervision	Requiring only standby assistance or verbal prompting or help with set-up
4	Minimal assistance	Requiring incidental hands-on help only (subject performs >75% of the task)
3	Moderate assistance	Subject still performs 50–75% of the task
2	Maximal assistance	Subject provides less than half of the effort (25–49%)
1	Total assistance	Subject contributes <25% of the effort or is unable to do the task

	The Functional Assessment Measure (FAM) includes FIM items but also adds 12 new items, covering cognition, such as community integration, emotional status, orientation, attention, reading and writing skills, and employability. A total score is given and can be used to illustrate added value across a client population. Client-level changes illustrating incremental change per task can be seen by using a 'FAM splat' visual diagram (Turner-Stokes et al., 2012). The UK FIM + FAM should be scored as a team, and record what the person does and not what they can do, when considering the preceding 24 hours. It can sometimes take about an hour to score; but as the team gains familiarity, scoring will take less time. Scorings can be repeated reliably across services.
Administration *For example, set-up* *and scoring, training* *requirements*	The scale can be administered by a physician, nurse, therapist or layperson as long as they have received training to use the measure correctly. Training involves attending a 1-day training course and subsequent practices.
Key references	Hamilton et al. (1987) and Turner-Stokes et al. (1999b, 2012)

Care needs and dependency level measures

Outcomes on the Barthel Index and the UK FIM + FAM are shown to correlate with care hours (Turner-Stokes et al., 1999b), but do not assess the number of people required to help nor the time taken to complete the task. This led to the development of The Northwick Park Dependency Score (NPDS) (Turner-Stokes et al., 1998) and the Northwick Park Care Needs Assessment (NPCNA) (Nyein and Turner-Stokes, 1999; Turner-Stokes et al., 1999a) both designed to provide an assessment on care hours and costs for clients at the more dependent end of the spectrum.

Both measures are observer-based activity-level measures and provide a numerical score that is then converted into hours of care/no of people required to assist. Both measures take about 10 minutes to complete, no training is required and can be repeated to show added value of therapy intervention at a client level or a client population level.

6.5.2 Commonly used impairment-level measures

The environment in which an occupational therapist works and their role within the team will often dictate the level of intervention that is used on a day-to-day basis. Although all occupational therapists should be familiar with occupational performance and ADL-level measures, knowledge of and confidence in using impairment-level measures is valuable and often required.

The following is a brief overview of impairment-level measures commonly seen in neurological rehabilitation (Tables 6.5 and 6.6).

6.5.3 Perceived health and QOL measure

Over the past 5 years or so, the biggest area of measurement development has been around the production of patient-reported outcome measures (PROMs). This trend has been driven by the need to demonstrate client choice over treatment, and the inclusion of PROMs is now seen as fundamental to inform the commissioning of services for a client population.

This has led to a huge expansion in the development of questionnaires, interview schedules and rating scales that measure states of health and illness from the client's perspective. PROMs allow clients to give feedback about the way they perceive their health and the impact that treatments or adjustments to lifestyle have on their QOL.

The list given in the text includes some more-established and well-used tools used to report QOL and other generic PROMs that elicit perceived day-to-day issues for clients and their carers (Table 6.7). In subsequent sections, disease-specific PROMs will be introduced to illustrate how PROMs can be used to highlight key issues around health, disease progression and QOL.

6.6 Disease-specific measures

Most of the following disease-specific measures were initially developed to help evaluate intervention within a research world. Increasing in popularity, most are now used in day-to-day practice by clinical teams and are often viewed as critical in demonstrating the impact of rehabilitation to support ongoing service funding. The reader should note that the world of outcome measurement is dynamic and more measures are being developed by clinical teams, particularly those related to disease-specific heath and illness.

The following section will introduce key measures used for clients with the four main progressive neurological diseases considered within this book:

Table 6.5 Physical impairment measures.

Name of measure	Measures	Brief description	Indicated reading
Motricity Index	Motor skills	A simple short and sensitive measure of motor skills. Validated for use in stroke but can be used for other upper motor neurone weakness.	Collin and Wade (1990) and Demeurisse et al. (1980)
Rivermead Mobility Index	Mobility	Simple to use, clinically relevant and reliable. Performance over 15 physical skills including lying, sitting, transfers, walking, stairs with the client reporting yes – 1, no – 0. The higher the score, the more physically able the client is.	Collen et al. (1990)
Timed 'up and go' (TUG) test	Sit to stand	The TUG test is a very easy-to-use test of sitting and standing balance plus mobility. The time it takes the client to rise from a chair, walk 3 m, turn around, walk back to the chair and sit down is timed and compared against norms. Developed for frail elderly, this measure has seen increasing popularity in Parkinson's rehabilitation research.	Morris et al. (2001) and Podsiadlo and Richardson (1991)
Berg Balance test	Balance	Fourteen-item scale designed to measure balance. Balance tasks get increasingly more difficult from sitting to standing, standing with eyes closed, standing on one foot. A 5-point scale from 0 to 4 gives a possible score out of 56, and a high/medium/low classification to predict the likelihood of falls. A change of 8 points is required to reveal a genuine change in function between two assessments.	Berg et al. (1989)
Ten-meter timed walk test	Cadence	Easy to set up and standardise, clients are asked to walk along a 10-m walkway while the therapist records total time taken and number of steps taken.	Bohannon and Andrews (1990) and Bradstater et al. (1983)
Modified Ashworth Scale (MAS)	Spasticity	Tests resistance to passive movement about a joint with varying degrees of velocity. The original Ashworth scores range from 0 to 4, with five choices. A score of 1 indicates no resistance and 5 indicates rigidity. The MAS adds a 1+ scoring category to indicate resistance through less than half of the movement. Thus the scores range gives six choices from 0, 1, 1+, 2, 3, 4. Once practised, the MAS is quick and reliable to use.	Ansari et al. (2008) and Bohannon and Smith (1987)
Nine-Hole Peg test	Dexterity	NHPT is a simple timed test of dexterity that involves the subjects placing nine dowels in nine holes. Subjects are set up in a standardised way and timed on removing and subsequently replacing nine dowels. Times are presented as standard deviation away from a norm.	Mathiowetz et al. (1985)
Action Research Arm Test (ARAT)	Upper limb	ARAT has four subsections of grasp, grip, pinch and gross movement are scored. Each subsection has incrementally challenging tasks that are passed or failed.	De Weerdt and Harrison (1985)
Visual Analogue Scales	Pain	Visual analogue scales and Numeric Graphic Rating Scales (where numbers are also added) are client-based measuring tools that can be used to answer a variety of questions ranging from level of pain to level of satisfaction with care. Pictorial pain scales have shown to be useful for clients with communication disorders and cognitive impairments.	Jackson et al. (2006)

Table 6.6 Cognitive impairment measures.

Name of measure	Measures	Brief description	Indicated reading
Test of Everyday Attention (TEA)	Attention	TEA uses eight subtests to explore attentional function, largely using everyday materials. Use of real-life scenarios means that clients enjoy the test and find it relevant to the problems faced in life. It is sensitive and clinically useful. The test takes about an hour to perform, and online training is required to learn to use the test.	Evans and Preston (2011)
Behavioural Assessment of Dysexecutive Syndrome (BADS)	Executive functioning	BADS specifically assesses the skills and demands involved in everyday life. It is sensitive to the capacities affected by frontal lobe damage, testing skills exercised in everyday situations. The test takes about an hour to perform, and online training is required to learn to use the test.	Wilson et al. (1998)
Doors and People	Long-term memory	Doors and People is a memory test that consists of four main categories: doors, people, shapes and names testing visual recognition, visual recall, verbal recognition and verbal recall. The test takes about 45 minutes to perform, and online training is required to learn to use the test.	Baddeley et al. (1994)
Hospital Anxiety and Depression Scale (HADS)	Mood	HADS was originally developed to be used by doctors to determine the levels of anxiety and depression that a client was experiencing. The HADS is a 14-item scale that generates ordinal data. Seven of the items relate to anxiety and seven relate to depression. Although superseded by many more specific assessment of mood, HADS is still frequently used in clinical practice.	Zigmond and Snaith (1983)

Table 6.7 Commonly used quality of life measures.

Name of measure	Measures	Brief description	Indicated reading
12-Item General Health Questionnaire (GHQ12)	Self-reported screen for well-being (general population)	The GHQ-12 is an extensively used instrument used to screen for mental health well-being in a general adult population. It is short (12 questions) and is used often to screen within populations of clients with long-term conditions as a first red flag for anxiety and depression. Self-reported by the client, the GHQ12 can be sent through the post and completed in 10 minutes.	Rickards (2005)
Medical Outcome Study Short Form (SF 36)	Self-reported screen for well-being (general population)	The SF-36 consists of 36 items split into 8-scaled scores that look at various aspects of health and well-being. Each scale is directly transformed into a 0 to 100 scale with a lower score indicating more disability. To calculate the scores, it is necessary to purchase special software. Its abbreviated version SF-6D is often used to evaluate health economics and the cost of disease burden.	Ware and Sherbourne (1992)

(continued)

Table 6.7 (Continued)

Name of measure	Measures	Brief description	Indicated reading
EUROQOL (EQ-5D)	Self-reported screen for well-being (general population)	The EQ-5D health questionnaire provides a simple descriptive profile and a single index value for health status. Increasing in international popularity, the EQ-5D is used to commission NHS services as it can be used to estimate quality-adjusted life years (QALYs). To note, there are numerous variations of this measure and specific software is used to provide results.	Dolan (1997)
NeuroQOL	Self-reported screen for well-being in neurologically impaired	NeuroQOL looks at health-related QOL in 17 domains and sub-domains. The measure requires no training to use and can be administered via Computer-Assisted Testing or in short forms. Each sub-domain that can be selected and administered separately depending upon individual client needs. The score generated gives a standard deviation away from the norm.	Cella et al. (2012)
Caregiver Strain Index	Perceived carer burden (general population)	The Caregiver Strain Index was one of the first means of identifying how the carer of the disabled client was coping. Although now superseded by disease specific care giver tools, the Caregiver Strain Index is still used frequently and has face validity and ease of utility.	Adelman et al. (2014) and Robinson (1983)

Table 6.8 Key measures for Huntington's disease.

Name of measure	Measures	Brief description	Indicated reading
Unified Huntington's Disease Rating Scale (UHDRS)	Impairment and activity level	The UHDRS is a tool developed to provide a uniform assessment of the clinical features and course of HD. Still mostly used in clinical research, the components of the UHDRS are as follows: **1** Motor Assessment **2** Cognitive Assessment **3** Behavioural Assessment **4** Independence Scale **5** Functional Assessment **6** Total Functional Capacity (TFC).	Huntington's Study Group (1996)
HD Health-Related QOL Questionnaire (HDQOL)	Self-reported QOL	HDQOL is a standardised instrument for measuring health-related QOL and is a validated disease-specific measure designed for HD. A summary score plus scores on several discrete scales indicates health-related QOL.	Hocaoglu et al. (2012)

Huntington's disease or HD (Table 6.8), *Motor neurone disease or MND* (Table 6.9), *multiple sclerosis or MS* (Table 6.10) *and Parkinson's* (Table 6.11). The measures included may be used by any member of the team including occupational therapists.

Table 6.9 Key measures for motor neurone disease.

Name of measure	Measures	Brief description	Indicated reading
Neurological Fatigue Index for MND (NFI-MND)	Fatigue	The NFI-MND is a simple, easy-to-administer 8-item fatigue scale. It includes separate scales for measuring fatigue experienced as reversible muscular weakness and fatigue expressed as feelings of low energy and whole-body tiredness.	Gibbons et al. (2011)
Amyotrophic Lateral Sclerosis Assessment Questionnaire (ALSAQ-40)	Self-reported quality of life (QOL)	The ALSQ-40 is a self-reported 40 point scale looking at the impact on MND on QOL. Compared to other non-MND-focused measures, the ALSAQ-40 covers areas related to psychological and spiritual issues.	Epton et al. (2009)
Herth Hope Index	Self-reported QOL-related to future hope	The Herth Hope Index is a quick and simple tool used to capture self-reported hope for people at the end of their life. Clients are asked to respond to 12 prewritten questions regarding quality of life and hope for the future being experienced now, using a 4-point Likert scale: strongly agree, agree, disagree, strongly disagree.	Herth (1992)
Edinburgh Cognitive and Behavioural ALS Screen (ECAS)	Cognitive impairment	The ECAS is a practical screening tool that incorporates a range of short cognitive tests that have shown to be sensitive to cognitive impairment in ALS.	Abrahams et al. (2014)

Table 6.10 Key measures for multiple sclerosis.

Name of measure	Measures	Brief description	Indicated reading
Expanded Disability Status Scale (EDSS)	Impairment-level measure	The EDSS is a method of quantifying disability in multiple sclerosis and monitoring changes in the level of disability over time. Scales from 0 to 5 or 0 to 6 are used to best describe body-level change in seven categories: **1** Visual function **2** Brainstem function **3** Pyramidal function **4** Cerebellar function **5** Sensory function **6** Bowel and bladder function **7** Cerebral function plus an ambulation score. The greater the score, the greater the body-level impairment and impact on functional mobility.	Kurtzke (1983)
Modified Fatigue Impact Scale	Self-reported impact of fatigue on activity and participation	The MFIS is a modified form of the FIS based on items derived from interviews with clients with MS concerning how fatigue impacts their lives. The full version consists of 21 items, whilst an abbreviated version with five items can also be used. This MFIS assesses the effects of fatigue in terms of physical, cognitive, and psychosocial functioning and is also included in the MSQLI.	Fisk et al. (1994)

(continued)

Table 6.10 (Continued)

Name of measure	Measures	Brief description	Indicated reading
MS Impact Scale – 29 (MSIS-29)	Self-reported quality of life (QOL)	MSIS-29 measures 20 physical items and 9 psychological impact of multiple sclerosis. Clients are asked to answer 29 questions about the impact of MS on their day-to-day life during the previous 2 weeks. The MSIS-29 has been found to be a clinically useful and scientifically sound client-based outcome measure of the impact of MS.	Hobart et al. (2005) and Riazi et al. (2002)
MS Quality of Life Inventory (MSQLI)	Self-reported QOL	The MSQLI is a battery consisting of 10 individual scales providing a QOL measure that is both generic and MS-specific. If all 10 self-reported questionnaires are competed, it takes about 45 minutes.	Fischer et al. (1999)

Table 6.11 Key measures for Parkinson's.

Name of measure	Measures	Brief description	Indicated reading
Hoehn and Yahr Staging	Impairment-level description	The Hoehn and Yahr scale was originally published in 1967, although still commonly used. It is a 5-point rating system for describing how the symptoms of Parkinson's progress.	Hoehn and Yahr (1967)
Unified Parkinson's disease rating scale (UPDRS)	Disease progression and disability	The UPDRS is a rating tool used to follow the longitudinal course of Parkinson's. It is made up of four parts: 1. Non-motor experiences of daily living split into two parts 1a – behaviours assessed by the investigator with information from the client and caregivers 1b – for completion by the client with the help of caregivers if desired, but independently of the investigator 2. Motor experiences of daily living – for completion by the client and/or caregivers as per 1b 3. Motor examination 4. Motor complications	Fahn et al. (1987) and Goetz et al. (2008)
Parkinson's Disease Questionnaire (PDQ 39 or PDQ 8)	Self-reported quality of life (QOL)	The PDQ-39 is a 39-item self-report questionnaire, which assesses Parkinson's-specific health-related quality over the last month. The PDQ-36 and its shorter version the PDQ-8 assess how often clients experience difficulties across the eight QOL dimensions looking at the impact of PD on specific dimensions of functioning and well-being. Easy to administrate and use.	Peto et al. (1998)

Information about measures and their use can be readily found on associated charities and support group websites. Clients can also be directed to find more information about the use and impact of measures in informing their care.

Case scenarios

Sarah was a 48-year-old lady with secondary progressive MS. She was reviewed in an out-patient MS disability clinic by the MS Clinical Nurse Specialist who completed the **MS Impact Scale - 19 (MSIS-19).** The MSIS-19 indicated that performance at home was beginning to change, and the occupational therapist then undertook an **Assessment of Motor and Process Skills (AMPS)** at home.

Lower limb tone and spasms were identified as one of the key issues impacting on motor skills during the AMPs, and the physiotherapist used the **Modified Ashworth Scale** to capture the extent of problems prior to developing a management plan. Some suggestion of declining executive skills was also seen during the process skills of the AMPS, and a subsequent assessment of problem-solving and executive functions was undertaken using the **Behavioural Assessment of the Dysexecutive Syndrome (BADS).**

Bill was a 72-year-old gentleman with Parkinson's who had a history of increasing falls over the last 2 months. He had been admitted to the Planned Investigation Unit for 4 days for a full medication review.

In order to identify what may be contributing to his falls, the **Timed-up-and-go (TUG) test** was completed by physiotherapist identifying increasing problems with trunk rotation. **The Unified Parkinson's Disease Rating Scale (UPDRS)** was also completed by the occupational therapist and some cognitive issues were raised. Bill was then seen by both the physiotherapist and occupational therapist at home and the **Canadian Occupational Performance Measure (COPM)** used to identify priority areas to address with Bill to increase his safety and satisfaction with performance at home.

Norman was a 62-year-old gentleman with a recent diagnosis of MND. Norman was still working full time but beginning to experience some problems.

The occupational therapist undertook the **COPM** in the MND MDT out-patient clinic and physical effort during morning routine was raised as an issue, which was impacting on the rest of Norman's day. The COPM showed that ease of access to a modified computer for work and energy available for leisure were priority areas to address and the occupational therapist completed the **Neurological Fatigue Index for MND (NFI-MND)** prior to setting up a full fatigue management programme with Norman.

Emotional adjustment to rapid loss was flagged up during the COPM, and the Regional Care Lead used the **Amyotrophic Lateral Sclerosis Assessment Questionnaire (ALSAQ-40)** to look at health-related QOL issues.

Sylvia was a 59-year-old lady with an 8-year history of HD. The occupational therapist was asked to see Sylvia at home by Social Worker as her husband was finding it increasingly difficult to cope despite having four daily visits from carers.

Sylvia was unable to reliably follow any formal instruction so the **Barthel ADL Index** was completed to baseline physical skills, following observation of Sylvia and discussion with her husband. The **Carer Giver Strain Index** was then completed by Sylvia's husband and used to highlight issues and facilitate initial discussions around increasing care at home to support Sylvia and her husband or consider the option of residential placement in the near future.

6.7 Self-evaluation questions

1 Do you understand the need to measure in your clinical area?
2 Can you recognise the components of good measure design?
3 Can you explain what a 'ceiling or floor effect' is in measurement?
4 Do you always identify your clinical question before measuring?
5 Which measures do you currently use within your practice?
6 Do you have an understanding of what your peers are using as their measures?
7 Can you explain the value of patient-reported outcome measures?
8 Do you routinely assess perceived burden for care-givers?
9 Do you have an awareness of the disease-specific measures you might need to use?
10 Can you describe how your measurement practice might change as the clients disease progresses?

References

Abrahams S, Newton J, Niven EH, Foley J and Bak THB (2014) Screening for cognitive and behaviour changes in ALS. Amyotrophic Lateral Sclerosis and Frontotemporal Degenerations. 15(1–2):9–14. doi:10.3109/21678421.2013.805784.

Adelman RD, Tmanova LL, Delgado D, Dion S and Lachs MS (2014) Caregiver burden: a clinical review. Care of the aging patient: from evidence to action. JAMA, 311(10):1052–1060.

Ansari NN, Naghdi S, Arab TK and Jalaie S (2008) The interrater and intrarater reliability of the Modified Ashworth Scale in the assessment of muscle spasticity: limb and muscle group effect. NeuroRehabilitation, 23(3):231–237.

Baddeley AD, Emslie H and Nimmo-Smith I (1994) Doors and people: a test of visual and verbal. Recall and recognition. Bury St. Edmunds: Thames Valley Test Company.

Berg K, Wood-Dauphinée S, Williams J and Gayton D (1989) Measuring balance in the elderly: preliminary development of an instrument. Physiotherapy Canada, 41(6):304–311.

Bohannon RW and Andrews AW (1990) Correlation of knee extensor muscle torque and spasticity with gait speed in patient with stroke. Archives of Physical Medicine and Rehabilitation, 71:330–333.

Bohannon R and Smith M (1987) Interrater reliability of a Modified Ashworth Scale of muscle spasticity. Physical Therapy, 67:206–220.

Bradstater ME, De Bruin H, Gowland C and Clarke BM (1983) Hemiplegic gait: analysis of temporal variables. Archives of Physical Medicine and Rehabilitation, 64:583–587.

British Society of Rehabilitation Medicine (2005) Measurement of outcome in rehabilitation. London: British Society of Rehabilitation Medicine, c/o Royal College of Physicians. Available at http://www.bsrm.co.uk/publications/BasketOfScoresWithSCIA%20_2_update2005newref9.pdf (Accessed 24 April 15).

Cella D, Lai JS, Nowinski CJ, Victorson D, Peterman A, Miller D, Bethoux F, Heinemann A, Rubin S, Cavazos JE, Reder AT, Sufit R, Simuni T, Holmes GL, Siderowf A, Wojna V, Bode R, McKinney N, Podrabsky T, Wortman K, Choi S, Gershon R, Rothrock N and Moy C (2012) Neuro-QOL: brief measures of health-related quality of life for clinical research in neurology. Neurology, 78(23):1860–1867.

College of Occupational Therapists (2012) Research briefing: measuring outcomes. London: College of Occupational Therapists.

Collen FM, Wade DT, Robb GF and Bradshaw CM (1990) The Rivermead Mobility Index: a further development of the Rivermead Motor Assessment. Disability and Rehabilitation, 13(2):50–54.

Collin C and Wade DT (1990) Assessing motor impairment after stroke: a pilot reliability study. Journal of Neurology, Neurosurgery, and Psychiatry, 53:576–579.

Collin C, Wade DT, Davis S and Horne V (1988) The Barthel ADL Index: a reliability study. International Disability Studies, 10:61–63.

De Weerdt W and Harrison MA (1985) Measuring recovery of arm-hand function in stroke patients: a comparison of the Brunnstrom-Fugl-Meyer test and the Action Research Arm test. Physiotherapy Canada, 37:65–70.

Dedding C, Cardol M, Eyssen IC, Dekker J and Beelen A (2004) Validity of the Canadian Occupational Performance Measure: a client-centred outcome measurement. Clinical Rehabilitation, 18(6):660–667.

Demeurisse G, Demol O and Robaye E (1980) Motor evaluation in vascular hemiplegia. European Neurology, 19:382–389.

Dolan P (1997) Modelling valuations in EuroQol health states. Medical Care, 35:1095–1108.

Epton J, Harris R and Jenkinson C (2009) Quality of life in amyotrophic lateral sclerosis/motor neuron disease: a structured review. Amyotrophic Lateral Sclerosis, 10:15–26.

Evans AS and Preston AS (2011) Test of everyday attention. In Encyclopedia of clinical neuro-psychology. London: Springer, pp. 2491–2492.

Fahn S, Elton R and Members of the UPDRS Development Committee (1987) The Unified Parkinson's Disease Rating Scale. In Fahn S, Marsden C, Calne D, Goldstein M (Eds) Recent developments in Parkinson's disease. Florham Park, NJ: Macmillan Healthcare Information, pp. 153–163.

Fawcett AL (2013) Principles of assessment and outcome measurement for occupational therapists and physiotherapists: theory, skills and application. Chichester: John Wiley & Sons, Ltd.

Fischer JS, Larocca, NG, Miller DM, Ritvo PG, Andrews H and Paty D (1999) Recent developments in the assessment of quality of life in multiple sclerosis (MS). Multiple Sclerosis Journal, 5(4):251–259.

Fisher AG (1994) Development of a functional assessment that adjusts ability measures for task simplicity and rater leniency. In Wilson M (Ed.) Objective measurement: theory into practice, Vol. 2. Norwood, NJ: Ablex, pp. 145–175.

Fisher AG (1997) Multifaceted measurement of daily life task performance: conceptualizing a test of instrumental ADL and validating the addition of personal ADL tasks. Physical Medicine and Rehabilitation: State of the Art Reviews, 11:289–303.

Fisher AG and Bray Jones K (2010a) Assessment of motor and process skills. Vol. 1: development, standardization, and administration manual, 7th Edition. Fort Collins, CO: Three Star Press.

Fisher AG and Bray Jones K (2010b) Assessment of motor and process skills. Vol. 2: user manual, 7th Edition. Fort Collins, CO: Three Star Press.

Fisk JD, Ritvo PG, Ross L, Haase DA, Marrie TJ and Schlech WF (1994) Measuring the functional impact of fatigue: initial validation of the fatigue impact scale. Clinical Infectious Diseases, 18(Suppl 1):S79–S83.

Gibbons C, Mills RJ, Thornton EW, Ealing J, Mitchell JD, Shaw PJ, Talbot K, Tennant A and Young CA (2011) Development of a patient reported outcome measure for fatigue in motor neurone disease: the Neurological Fatigue Index (NFI-MND). Health and Quality of Life Outcomes, 9:101.

Goetz CG, Tilley BC, Shaftman SR, Stebbins GT, Fahn S, Martinez-Martin P, Poewe W, Sampaio C, Stern MB, Dodel R, Dubois B, Holloway R, Jankovic J, Kulisevsky J, Lang AE, Lees A, Leurgans S, LeWitt PA, Nyenhuis D, Olanow CW, Rascol O, Schrag A, Teresi JA, van Hilten JJ, LaPelle N; Movement Disorder Society UPDRS Revision Task Force (2008) Movement disorder society-sponsored revision of the unified Parkinson's disease rating scale (MDS-UPDRS): scale presentation and clinimetric testing results. Movement Disorders, 23(15):2129–2170.

Hamilton BB, Granger CV, Sherwin FS, Zielezny M and Tashman JS (1987) A uniform national data system for medical rehabilitation. In Fuhrer JM (Ed.) Rehabilitation outcomes: analysis and measurement. Baltimore, MD: Brookes, pp. 137–147.

Herth K (1992) Abbreviated instrument to measure hope: development and psychometric evaluation. Journal of Advanced Nursing, 17:1251–1259.

Hobart J, Riazi A, Lamping D, Fitzpatrick R and Thompson A (2005) How responsive is the Multiple Sclerosis Impact Scale (MSIS-29)? A comparison with some other self-report scales. Journal of Neurology, Neurosurgery, and Psychiatry, 76(11):1539–1543.

Hocaoglu MB, Gaffan EA and Ho AK (2012) The Huntington's disease Health-Related Quality of Life questionnaire (HDQoL): a disease-specific measure of health-related quality of life. Clinical Genetics, 81(2):117–122.

Hoehn M and Yahr M (1967) Parkinsonism: onset, progression and mortality. Neurology, 17(5):427–442.

Holbrook M and Skilbeck CE (1983) An activities index for use with stroke patients. Age and Ageing, 12:166–170.

Huntington's Study Group (1996) The Unified Huntington's Disease Rating Scale: reliability and consistency. Movement Disorders, 11:136–142.

Jackson D, Horn S, Kersten P and Turner-Stokes L (2006) Development of a pictorial scale of pain intensity for patients with communication impairments: initial validation in a general population. Clinical Medicine, 6(6):580–585.

Kielhofner G (2002) A model of human occupation: theory and application. Philadelphia, PA: Lippincott Williams & Wilkins.

Kurtzke JF (1983) Rating neurologic impairment in multiple sclerosis: an expanded disability status scale (EDSS). Neurology, 33(11):1444–1452.

Law M, Baptiste S, McColl M, Opzoomer A, Polatajko H and Pollock N (1990) The Canadian occupational performance measure: an outcome measure for occupational therapy. Canadian Journal of Occupational Therapy [Revue Canadienne d Ergotherapie], 57(2):82–87.

Law M, Baptiste S, Carswell A, McColl MA, Polatajko H and Pollock N (2005) Canadian occupational performance measure, 4th Edition. Ottawa, ON: Canadian Association of Occupational Therapists. www.thecopm.ca/.

Mahoney FI and Barthel DW (1965) Functional evaluation: the Barthel Index. Maryland State Medical Journal, 14:61–65.

Mathiowetz V, Weber K, Kashman N and Volland G (1985) Adult norms for the Nine Hole Peg Test of finger dexterity. Occupational Therapy Journal of Research, 5:24–37.

Morris S, Morris M and Iansek R (2001) Reliability of measurements obtained with the Timed 'Up and Go' test in people with Parkinson disease. Physical Therapy, 81(2):810–818.

Nouri FM and Lincoln NB (1987) An extended activities of daily living scale for stroke patients. Clinical Rehabilitation, 1:301–305.

Nyein K and Turner-Stokes L (1999) Sensitivity and predictive value of the Northwick Park Care Needs Assessment (NPCNA) as a measure of care needs in the community. Clinical Rehabilitation, 13(6):482–491.

Parkinson S, Forsyth K and Kielhofner G (2006) The Model of Human Occupation Screening Tool (MOHOST) version 2.0. University of Illinois Board of Trustees. Available at http://www.cade.uic.edu/moho/products.aspx (Accessed 27 April 2015).

Peto V, Jenkinson C and Fitzpatrick R (1998) PDQ-39: a review of the development, validation and application of a Parkinson's disease quality of life questionnaire and its associated measures. Journal of Neurology, 245(Suppl 1):S10–S14.

Podsiadlo D and Richardson S (1991) The Timed 'Up and Go': a test of basic functional mobility for frail elderly persons. Journal of the American Geriatrics Society, 39(2):142–148.

Riazi A, Hobart JC, Lamping DL, Fitzpatrick R and Thompson AJ (2002) Multiple Sclerosis Impact Scale (MSIS-29): reliability and validity in hospital based samples. Journal of Neurology, Neurosurgery, and Psychiatry, 73(6):701–704.

Rickards H (2005) Depression in neurological disorders: Parkinson's disease, multiple sclerosis and stroke. Journal of Neurology, Neurosurgery, and Psychiatry, 76:i48–i52.

Robinson BC (1983) Validation of a caregiver strain index. Journal of Gerontology, 38:344–348.

Turner-Stokes L, Tonge P, Nyein K, Hunter M, Nielson S and Robinson I (1998) The Northwick Park Dependency Score (NPDS): a measure of nursing dependency in rehabilitation. Clinical Rehabilitation, 12(4):304–318.

Turner-Stokes L, Nyein K and Halliwell D (1999a) The Northwick Park Care Needs Assessment (NPCNA): a directly costable outcome measure in rehabilitation. Clinical Rehabilitation, 13(3): 253–267.

Turner-Stokes L, Nyein K, Turner-Stokes T and Gatehouse C (1999b) The UK FIM+FAM: development and evaluation. Functional Assessment Measure. Clinical Rehabilitation, 13(4):277–287.

Turner-Stokes L, Williams H, Sephton K, Rose H, Harris S and Thu A (2012) Engaging the hearts and minds of clinicians in outcome measurement – the UK Rehabilitation Outcomes Collaborative approach. Disability and Rehabilitation, 34(22):1871–1879.

UK Rehabilitation Outcomes Collaborative (2015) Clinical tools: complexity of needs, clinical tools and outcome measures. London: Kings College London. http://www.kcl.ac.uk/lsm/research/divisions/cicelysaunders/research/studies/ukroc/tools.aspx (Accessed 24 February 15).

Wade DT and Collin C (1988) The Barthel ADL Index: a standard measure of physical disability? International Disability Studies, 10(2):64–67.

Ware JE and Sherbourne CD (1992) The MOS 36-item Short-Form Health Survey (SF-36): I. Conceptual framework and item selection. Medical Care, 30:473–483.

Wilson BA, Evans JJ, Emslie H, Alderman N and Burgess P (1998) The development of an ecologically valid test for assessing patients with a dysexecutive syndrome. Neuropsychological Rehabilitation, 8:213–228.

Zigmond AS and Snaith RP (1983) The hospital anxiety and depression scale. Acta Psychiatrica Scandinavica, 67(6):361–370.

CHAPTER 7
Occupational therapy intervention

7.1 Introduction

Occupational therapists offer a range of interventions and management strategies to support people living with long-term neurological conditions to maximise their existing skills and resources and to support successful engagement in meaningful occupations. This can include a range of practical, occupation-focussed interventions and behavioural approaches aimed at changing maladaptive responses into positive approaches which support the person living with a long-term neurological condition to maximise opportunities for engagement and wider participation. This chapter explores a range of rehabilitative interventions to support the occupational therapist to work collaboratively with the person living with a long-term neurological condition to achieve their occupational goals.

7.1.1 Rehabilitation interventions

Rehabilitation is defined as 'a set of measures that assist individuals, who experience or are likely to experience disability, to achieve and maintain optimum functioning in interaction with their environments' (World Health Organisation, 2011). Rehabilitation aims 'through peer support, to enable persons with disabilities to attain and maintain their maximum independence, full physical, mental, social and vocational ability, and full inclusion and participation in all aspects of life' (von Groote et al., 2011).

Rehabilitation measures are aimed at achieving the following broad outcomes (World Health Organisation, 2012):

- Prevention of the loss of function
- Slowing the rate of loss of function
- Improvement or restoration of function
- Compensation for lost function
- Maintenance of current function.

Occupational Therapy and Neurological Conditions, First Edition. Edited by Jenny Preston and Judi Edmans.
© 2016 John Wiley & Sons, Ltd. Published 2016 by John Wiley & Sons, Ltd.

7.2 Activities of daily living

The term 'activities of daily living' is used to describe fundamental aspects of self-care which are performed as part of our everyday routines. Symptoms such as pain, fatigue, weakness and balance can impact on the successful completion of activities including eating, dressing, bathing, toileting and grooming. The occupational therapist should consider a range of strategies which are relevant and appropriate to each individual person. Some general principles which can be applied to support activities of daily living include the following:

7.2.1 Dressing
- Lay out clothes before starting to get dressed and place them on the bed or a chair so that they are within easy reach avoiding unnecessary bending or stretching.
- Sit down to get dressed if balance is impaired.
- Apply all lower garments first before standing to adjust clothing. This minimises the need for repeated standing and conserves energy.
- Avoid tight-fitting garments if sitting for prolonged periods in a wheelchair.
- Use garments with elasticated waist for easier access for toileting.
- Avoid small fastenings, including buttons and zip fasteners.
- Avoid shoes with laces, choose slip-on shoes or Velcro fastenings.
- Cotton garments may be more comfortable than man-made fibres such as nylon or polyester.

7.2.2 Eating and drinking
- Ensure a good upright position can be maintained throughout mealtimes.
- Smaller portions may be easier to manage and prevents food from getting cold.
- Plate warming devices may help keep the food more appetising.
- If the person needs assistance to cut up food, this should be done discretely in advance of serving the meal.
- Non-slip mats, adapted cutlery and plate guards may help to manoeuvre the food onto a fork or spoon.
- Consider using a spoon instead of a fork.
- Avoid filling glasses and cups to prevent spilling if tremor is apparent.
- Two-handled mugs or heavier mugs may help reduce tremor.
- Electronic eating devices or mobile arm supports may assist with eating.
- Consider using thickeners in liquids if choking becomes apparent and refer to speech and language therapy for further advice.

7.2.3 Toileting
- Consider using fixed grab rails by the toilet.
- Avoid using free-standing toilet frames for people with Parkinson's or Huntington's (Aragon and Kings, 2010; Cook et al., unpublished) as the movement within them can interfere with safe transfers.

- Choreic movements or excessive force when sitting can lead to increased pressure on toilet seats which may break more frequently (Cook et al., unpublished).
- Use of washing and drying toilet facilities should be considered to promote personal hygiene.
- Garments which can be easily laundered should be considered when bladder and bowel problems exist.
- When bladder problems exist darker coloured clothing may be more discrete in the event of an 'accident'.

7.2.4 Bed mobility
- Teach methods for turning and rolling in bed.
- Consider using satin night-wear or bedclothes to aid movement in bed (Aragon and Kings, 2010).
- Use of additional pillows or foam wedges help maintain posture and prevent sliding.
- Encourage the person to get into bed by sitting on the edge of the bed near to the pillows and lifting legs into bed before lying down (Aragon and Kings, 2010).

7.2.5 Grooming
- Use of an electric shaver or beard trimmer is safer than a wet shave (Cook et al., unpublished).
- Shorter hairstyles are easier to manage, but for those people who wish to keep longer hair a 'tangle teaser' brush or spray-in conditioner helps to keep hair manageable (Cook et al., unpublished).

7.3 Fatigue management

Fatigue management incorporates a self-management approach to supporting the person living with a long-term neurological condition to increase their understanding of the factors contributing to or exacerbating fatigue and through education and adaptation learning to optimise their function (Harrison, 2007). Fatigue management can be applied at an individual level or can be carried out as a group activity, for example the FACETS (Fatigue: Applying Cognitive behavioural and Energy effectiveness Techniques to lifeStyle) programme (Thomas et al., 2010).

The key principles of fatigue management include the following:
- Education to develop an understanding of energy conservation strategies
- Generation of practical solutions including access to resources and equipment
- Development of strategies which challenge underlying health beliefs
- Increased activity and participation through collaborative goal setting.

7.3.1 Practical strategies for energy conservation

The following practical strategies for energy conservation have been adapted from Harrison (2007).

Take frequent rests
- Build in time for rest within and between everyday activities.
- Taking regular, short rests instead of one long rest, that is sitting down for 5 minutes while vacuuming a room instead of waiting until the room is completely vacuumed and then taking a 30-minute rest.

Prioritise activities
- List all the jobs which need to be done across the day/week.
- Delegate jobs which can be done by somebody else.
- Ask for help! Access help from others, including external agencies.
- Reduce or cut out jobs which may not be necessary, for example folding washing may prevent the need for ironing or avoid ironing items such as socks or towels.
- Consider how certain tasks are completed, for example washing small amounts everyday instead of a large wash once a week to spread out the amount of work.

Plan ahead
- Complete the most important tasks first to prevent running out of energy.
- Use schedules or plans of activities on a daily or weekly basis.
- Spread heavy and light tasks across the day.
- Don't be too ambitious! Set realistic targets.
- Try to avoid tasks which cannot be stopped should you feel tired.

Organise tools, materials and work area
- Organise work areas to reduce effort and unnecessary movements including bending.
- Ensure lighting is good to prevent eye strain.
- Think about the temperature of the room and try to avoid it becoming too hot.
- Organise areas to make sure that relevant items are close at hand, for example arrange cupboards to place most frequently used items at the front.
- Try to avoid clutter.

Adopt a good posture
- Try to reduce stress on the body, moving efficiently, avoiding twisting and bending.
- Maintain symmetry and an upright posture during tasks.
- Rest between repetitive tasks.

Lead a healthy lifestyle
- Choose activities that you enjoy.
- Use the correct equipment.
- Build up slowly to new activities.
- Plan exercise as part of daily/weekly routines.
- Eat a well-balanced diet.
- Avoid heavy meals.
- Remember that excess weight, alcohol and smoking can all have a negative effect on fatigue.

7.4 Cognitive rehabilitation

Cognitive rehabilitation can be described as any intervention strategy or technique which enables people living with a long-term neurological condition and their families or carers to live with, manage, by-pass, reduce or come to terms with cognitive deficits (Wilson, 1987). Cognitive rehabilitation utilises therapeutic activities in a systematic way to promote functional changes within the person's everyday life and also have a key role to play in occupational therapy practice (Worthington, 2007, p. 266).

Occupational therapy interventions aimed at cognitive rehabilitation tend to fall within the following two main categories of approach:

- The **adaptive approach** which focuses on making best use of residual skills and abilities. Use of the adaptive approach enables people with long-term neurological conditions to engage successfully within their chosen occupations through application of compensatory strategies, environmental adaptation or through learning new skills (Toglia et al., 2009). Examples of this could include using lists; apps on mobile phones and tablets, alarms and paging devices, and pill dispensers. Using technology to support participation is discussed more fully in Chapter 8.

- The **remedial or restorative approach** aims to reduce impairment by teaching the brain to re-learn or develop new ways of functioning. Stuifbergen et al. (2012) found evidence of improved verbal memory and increased frequency of using memory strategies in a sample of people with moderate cognitive impairment associated with multiple sclerosis (MS) following computer-based exercises.

Due to the progressive nature of their diseases, people living with a long-term neurological condition are often considered to be poor candidates for cognitive rehabilitation, but this should be considered within the selection of interventions to best meet the their needs (Brooks and Matson, 1982).

7.4.1 General principles of cognitive rehabilitation

- Interventions must be tailored to suit the individual.
- Interventions are most effective when developed collaboratively between the person living with a long-term neurological condition, their family and the occupational therapist.
- Interventions should be focussed on mutually set and functionally relevant goals.
- Evaluation of the efficacy and outcome should incorporate and capture changes in functional abilities.
- The most successful cognitive interventions involve multiple approaches.
- Interventions should recognise the person's awareness of their situation and their ability to self-regulate behaviour and emotion.
- Interventions should address the person's emotional response to cognitive challenges and their general coping style, for example getting angry or frustrated.
- Interventions should be self-evaluative, that is the person living with a long-term neurological condition needs to be able to determine if change or improvement has occurred.

7.4.2 General principles in the management of memory disorders

Encoding (the registration of information)
- Simplify the information.
- Reduce the amount of information.
- Make sure information is understood.
- Link/associate information, for example remember a shopping list by rooms in the house.
- Little and often rule.
- Encourage organisation.
- Process information at a deeper level, for example using emotional or visual connection with the information.

Storing
- Test/rehearse/practice.
- Use expanding rehearsal, that is begin with a small amount of information and learn it before adding another section.

Retrieval
- Present information in several different contexts such as questioning in a different way: Do you go out much? When do you go swimming? Is it Monday or Tuesday when you go swimming?
- First letter prompts, for example his name starts with 'J'.

- Alphabetical searching, for example when trying to remember items on a shopping list: apples, bread, cat food.
- Mental retracing, that is imagining being in the room or in the situation where the event occurred, for example mentally walking through each room in your house as you stand in the supermarket to remember what you need to buy. You then recall that as you were showering in the morning you ran out of shower gel.

7.4.3 Commonly used intervention strategies

Environmental interventions
- Labelling cupboard contents.
- Message centre on fridge door.
- Use of cues, for example note on door to remember keys.
- Use of checklists, for example dressing sequence.
- Organisation of physical space, for example keep free from clutter and distraction.

Compensatory devices and strategies
- Calendars.
- Alarm clocks.
- Mobile phones.
- Personal computers and tablets.
- Paging systems.

Specialised instruction techniques
- Mnemonics, for example **E**very **G**ood **B**oy **D**eserves **F**ood to learn musical notes.
- PQRST (Preview-Question-Read-State-Test) when reading, for example newspaper articles.
- Errorless learning.
- Direct instruction techniques.
- Procedural learning.

7.4.4 Generalisation

Generalisation or transfer of training refers to the application of a skill learned in one particular situation to a different but similar situation. Strategies which are used within one context may not apply within another, for example PQRST might help with reading short articles in the newspaper but not when reading longer chapters of a book. Similarly the person living with a long-term neurological condition may find that some strategies work well for a particular problem but not for others, for example mental retracing to remember a shopping list might not help with remembering names. Failure to generalise, however, does not mean that the intervention is not effective but that further discussion may be required between the occupational therapist and the person living with a long-term neurological condition to find the most appropriate solution.

7.5 Anxiety management

Anxiety is a feeling that is common to us all at some stage within our daily lives and is generally perceived as a natural reaction to certain situations and circumstances (SANE, 2015). For most people, this tends to pass relatively quickly without any interventions. However for some people living with a long-term neurological condition this can be become quite disabling and can interfere with daily life.

Diagnosis with a long-term neurological condition can lead to a fear or apprehension of what lies ahead or what the future might hold. Anxiety often goes hand-in hand with depression and can become a major barrier for some people living with a long-term neurological condition impacting on their ability to engage in their chosen occupations, their relationships and their interactions with their environment. Feelings of inadequacy and an inability to cope with the demands placed upon them can lead to challenges for the person living with a long-term neurological condition, their family and friends.

7.5.1 Symptoms of anxiety

Psychological effects of anxiety may include the following (SANE, 2015):
- An overwhelming sense of fearful anticipation
- Inability to concentrate
- Constant worrying
- Heightened alertness and a tendency to 'catastrophise'
- Sleep disturbance.
    Physical effects may include the following:
- Tightness in the chest, chest pains or a 'pounding' heart
- Nausea
- Rapid shallow breathing or butterfly feelings in the stomach
- Loss of appetite
- Headaches
- Dizziness or feeling faint
- Muscle tension
- Sweating
- Frequent urination
- Panic attacks.

7.5.2 Strategies for managing anxiety
Understanding anxiety

People understand anxiety in different ways, and this can impact on how they then choose to manage it. For some people living with a long-term neurological condition, anxiety serves as a protective function as they believe that by anticipating certain dangers they can recognise and avoid them or that they will be better prepared to cope with them. This can however lead to unnecessary worrying and the person living with a long-term neurological condition may begin to worry about the amount of time they spend worrying, becoming increasingly focussed on the symptoms of anxiety, which in turns adds to their worry. This focus on potential danger may also lead to the person living with a long-term neurological condition avoiding situations or disengagement in certain occupations.

Time use may also contribute to levels of anxiety as lack of time for relaxation can contribute to higher levels of anxiety. Conversely having too much time to dwell on potential dangers may mean that the person living with a long-term neurological condition has more opportunities to engage in worry and feel anxious (adapted from Moodjuice, 2015).

Challenging patterns of unhelpful thinking

It is common when living with a long-term neurological condition to spend a lot of time thinking about the future and predicting what could go wrong, for example 'I'll be using a wheelchair within 2 years'. For others they may make assumptions about other people's beliefs without any real evidence to support them, for example 'they think I'm drunk at 5 o'clock in the morning'. One of the main factors contributing to heightened anxiety for people living with a long-term neurological condition however is catastrophising or blowing things out of proportion, that is they assume that something that has happened is far worse than it really is, for example 'I won't get another occupational therapy appointment because I forgot about the last one', or they may think that something terrible is going to happen in the future, when in reality, there is very little evidence to support it, for example 'My children will be taken from me if I'm not able to look after them properly'.

People living with a long-term neurological condition may focus on the negatives or imagine how things ought to be, applying extra pressure on them to achieve perfection. Loss of confidence also contributes to anxiety and previous experiences or isolated incidents can lead to the person living with a long-term neurological condition worrying that the same thing will happen again, for example 'I went shopping with my friends and couldn't find a toilet. I spent all the time worrying in case I had an accident, so now I don't go shopping'. Attachment of negative labels by the person living with a long-term neurological condition can influence how they see themselves and can further heighten anxiety levels, for example 'I'm stupid', 'I'm useless' or 'I'm a burden to my family' (adapted from Moodjuice, 2015).

The occupational therapist can help the person living with a long-term neurological condition to recognise and challenge unhelpful thoughts. This is done by asking the following series of questions (adapted from Moodjuice, 2015):

1 Is there any evidence that contradicts this thought?
  - I've always been the one to support my family
  - I'm always there to look after my children
2 Can you identify any of the patterns of unhelpful thinking described earlier?
  - I see parents much worse than me and their children haven't been taken from them.
3 What would you say to a friend who had this thought in a similar situation?
  - I'd say, don't be ridiculous you are a great mother. You are always there for your children. As long as you look after your own health you should be fine. Besides, you can only do your best.
4 What are the costs and benefits of thinking in this way?
  - Costs: it's making me feel sick with worry
  - Benefits: I can't really think of any
5 How will you feel about this in 6 months?
  - I will still probably be worrying about how good a mother I am because that is the type of person I am. I never like to give myself credit for doing a good job.
6 Is there another way of looking at this situation?
  - I make sure that the children don't see me at my worst. I often rest when they are in school so that I have the energy to do things with them when they come home. Most parents get tired at some point.
7 Try to come up with a more balanced or rational view.
  - I've worried about this since the children were born and they seem to be doing okay, so far. I'm sure every parent worries about how they bring up their children but I just worry more because of my condition, which probably has nothing to do with how good a parent I am.

Problem solving

People living with a long-term neurological condition might find it more difficult to cope if they feel they have lots of problems that they can't seem to get on top of. This ultimately leads to worrying or ruminating over the problems without finding a way to resolve them, making the person living with a long-term neurological condition feel more upset or even interfere with their sleep. Use of a problem-solving approach can support the person living with a long-term neurological problem to clearly articulate and frame the problem, identify priorities and generate potential solutions to overcome the problem (adapted from Moodjuice, 2015). An example of applying a problem-solving approach might include (adapted from Moodjuice, 2015):

1 What is the problem? Try to be as specific as possible.
  - e.g. I won't be able to go shopping if I no longer have a driving license.
2 How have you solved similar problems in the past?
  - e.g. I used to get a lift from my friend/I used on-line shopping/I used public transport/my husband did the shopping on his way home from work

3 What would your friends or family advise?
- e.g. come with us when we go shopping and we can turn it into a day out/I always use on-line shopping now as I can do it any time of the day or night to suit my own needs/let your husband get on with it, he does nothing else to help!

4 How would you like to see yourself tackling this problem?
- e.g. I want to be able to continue to do the shopping as it helps me plan for the week and to keep an eye on how much money I am spending

5 Select the best solution from the list. Think carefully about each option and consider the 'for' and 'against' for each idea. This will help to make a good decision and select the best solution.
- e.g. I think I will start to shop online as I can still be in charge of what I am buying and I can do it at a time when I feel able to really concentrate on this.

Limiting the time spent worrying

Engagement in meaningful occupations can help the person living with a long-term neurological condition to make more effective use of their time subsequently reducing the amount of time available for worrying and reduce the level of anxiety. Allocating specific 'worry time' within their daily schedule may however be a useful practical strategy for some people living with a long-term neurological condition. This involves setting aside between 15 and 20 minutes each day in which the person 'allows' themselves to worry. They should be encouraged to write down any worries which pop into their head outside of the 'worry time' and forget about them until later that day when they will try to resolve them during the 'worry time'. By noting them down the person living with a long-term neurological condition can feel safe in the knowledge that the worries won't be forgotten about. This strategy aims to free up time during the day that is normally wasted worrying.

When the 'worry time' arrives the person living with a long-term neurological condition allows themselves to think about the things that have been worrying them during the day and attempts to resolve them. 'Worry time' not only reduces the amount of time spent worrying during the day with subsequent physical and emotional benefits for the person living with a long-term neurological condition but can also alter perceptions of having more control about engagement in worry or not. Returning to the worries at a later point in the day allows the person living with a long-term neurological condition to approach the worries with a 'fresh-eye' while many of the worries will have resolved themselves or simply seem less important (adapted from Moodjuice, 2015).

Relaxation

Techniques associated with relaxation can be helpful for anxiety disorders where psychological stress is a factor. There are a range of self-administered stress management and relaxation techniques which can be accessed by people living with a long-term neurological condition, for example listening to music, having a relaxing bath or watching a movie.

Mind–body approaches are often used by people with long-term neurological conditions with increasing evidence of their effectiveness (Senders et al., 2012). Mind–body approaches focus on the relationships between the brain, mind, body and behaviour and their effect on health and disease (Wahbeh et al., 2008). Commonly used techniques include mindfulness, meditation; relaxation and breathing techniques; visual imagery, yoga, tai chi, hypnotherapy and biofeedback.

The occupational therapist may require additional training to be able to deliver some of these techniques or may choose to refer the person living with a long-term neurological condition for more specialist support. However, occupational therapists will be able to facilitate controlled breathing, muscular relaxation and visual imagery techniques as follows:

Controlled breathing
- Get into a comfortable position.
- Work out a stable breathing rhythm.
- Breathe in for 3 seconds, hold this breathe for 2 seconds, and then breathe out for 3 seconds. It can be helpful to count, for example In: 1–2–3, HOLD: 1–2, Out: 1–2–3, HOLD: 1–2.
- Repeat this action for a few minutes until you begin to feel more relaxed (adapted from Moodjuice, 2015).

Muscular relaxation
- Find somewhere comfortable and quiet, free from interruptions.
- Sit or lie down.
- Begin by focussing on your breathing; try to develop a slow and comfortable pace.
- Do this for a few minutes to prepare for the muscular relaxation.
- Try to tense each muscle group for around 5 seconds. Don't tense the muscle too tight.
- Focus on the sensations this brings.
- Then relax your muscles for a similar length of time, and again, focus on how this feels.
- Then move on to the next muscle group.
- Try to keep your breathing at a comfortable pace throughout.
- Legs: point your toes and tense your muscles as if you were trying to stand up.
- Stomach: tense your stomach muscles.
- Arms: make fists and tense your muscles as if you were trying to lift something.
- Shoulders: shrug your shoulders. Lift them up towards your ears.

- Face: make a frowning expression. Squeeze your eyes and shut and screw up your nose. Clench your teeth.
- To complete the sequence, lie quietly in a relaxed state for a few minutes. See if you are aware of tension in your body and try to relax it. Otherwise just let the tension be. If your mind wanders, try to bring your concentration back to your breathing.
- Finally count down silently and slowly: 5–4–3–2–1–0 and come out of relaxation in your own time. Try to carry that feeling of relaxation into your next activity (adapted from Moodjuice, 2015).

Visual imagery
- Find a private calm space and make yourself comfortable.
- Take a few slow and deep breaths to centre your attention and calm yourself.
- Close your eyes.
- Imagine yourself in a beautiful location, where everything is as you would ideally have it. Some people visualise a beach, a mountain, a forest, or being in a favourite room sitting on a favourite chair.
- Imagine yourself becoming calm and relaxed. Alternatively, imagine yourself smiling, feeling happy and having a good time.
- Focus on the different sensory attributes present in your scene so as to make it more vivid in your mind. For instance, if you are imagining the beach, spend some time vividly imagining the warmth of the sun on your skin, the smell of the ocean, seaweed and salt spray, and the sound of the waves, wind and seagulls. The more you can invoke your senses, the more vivid the entire image will become.
- Remain within your scene, touring its various sensory aspects for 5–10 minutes or until you feel relaxed.
- While relaxed, assure yourself that you can return to this place whenever you want or need to relax.
- Open your eyes again and then re-join your world (adapted from Post-White and Fitzgerald, 2002).

Distraction
Engagement in meaningful occupations can serve as a distraction and help the person living with a long-term neurological condition to take their mind off their problems. However some simple strategies for distraction include the following: counting backwards from 1000 in multiples of 7; focus on breathing and how it feels to inhale and exhale; visual imagery, imagining oneself in a safe place; while listening to music, try to identify different instruments and sounds (adapted from Moodjuice, 2015).

Reducing avoidance

Use of avoidance strategies as a coping mechanism can contribute to heightened anxiety and the development of irrational fears or loss of confidence. The occupational therapist can facilitate the use of progressive exposure to a stimulus which provokes anxiety or other negative reaction, in a safe environment, until the person living with a long-term neurological condition can tolerate the stimulus without becoming dysfunctional (Hagedorn, 2001).

An example of this might be in relation to a person living with a long-term neurological condition who wants to go swimming with her children but who is afraid of being in the water. The occupational therapist would support the person living with a long-term neurological condition through a process which might involve the following:

1 Identifying the most suitable swimming pool based on accessibility, safety, supervision, etc.
2 Visit the swimming pool as a spectator only.
3 Identify opportunities for lessons or practical support.
4 Purchase or borrow swim aids.
5 Identify swimwear which feels comfortable.
6 First stage: sit at the edge of the pool and test the temperature and buoyancy of the water.
7 Second stage: enter the pool and stay close to the edge.
8 Third stage: gentle splashing of face with water.
9 Fourth stage: practice putting head under water.
10 Fifth stage: move from the edge of the pool.
11 Sixth stage: attempt to swim.

7.6 Falls management

Falls are a significant issue for people living with long-term neurological conditions with more than half reporting at least one fall within the last 12 months (Busse et al., 2009; Nilsagard et al., 2009; Stolze et al., 2004). People living with long-term neurological conditions are twice as likely to fall when compared to an age-matched community-dwelling population (Stolze et al., 2004). Increased falls risk is associated with impairments of cognition (Gunn et al., 2013); disorders affecting gait and balance; insufficient walking aids; environmental factors at home; fear of falling; and medication (Stolze et al., 2004).

Occupational therapy intervention, for people living with a long-term neurological condition who have fallen, are at risk of falling or who are fearful of falling, incorporates a range of strategies which include identification of risk factors, assessment of occupational performance, interventions and self-management strategies (College of Occupational Therapists, 2015).

7.6.1 Identification of people at risk

- The occupational therapist should routinely ask the person living with a long-term neurological condition if they have fallen in the past year.
- Details about the frequency, context and characteristics of the fall(s) should be established.
- The occupational therapist should ask about diet, medication, physical activity and cognition as triggers for increased risk of falling.

7.6.2 Assessment of occupational performance

- The occupational therapist should assess an individual's ability to perform activities of daily living that they need or wish to perform independently and safely (e.g. getting dressed, cooking a meal and walking outside); roles (e.g. returning to work and caring for another person); social and psychological considerations; cognition; fear; confidence; and mental capacity.

7.6.3 Interventions

Minimising risk

- Offer a home hazard assessment to people at risk of falls.
- Offer a home safety assessment and modification for people with a visual impairment.
- Offer information and instruction on assistive devices as part of a home hazard assessment.
- Enable the person living with a long-term neurological condition to minimise the risk of falling when engaging in meaningful occupations.
- Facilitate caregivers, family and friends to adopt a positive approach to risk taking.

Fear of falling

- Listen to the person's concerns about their falls risk and access objective assessments as appropriate.
- Develop an individualised plan, in collaboration with the person living with a long-term neurological condition, to promote engagement in meaningful occupations to overcome fear of falling.

Falls prevention

- Share knowledge and understanding of falls prevention and management strategies.
- Take into account the perceptions and beliefs of the person living with a long-term neurological condition regarding their ability and personal motivation which may influence participation in falls interventions.

- Maximise the extent to which the person living with a long-term neurological condition feels in control of the falls intervention.
- Support the engagement of the person living with a long-term neurological condition to identify positive benefits of falls intervention.
- Offer falls prevention and management information in different formats.
- Encourage participation in physical and social activity as a means of reducing risk of falls and their adverse consequences through the engagement in meaningful occupations.
- Offer activities to improve strength and balance that are meaningful to the person living with a long-term neurological condition to improve and encourage longer-term participation in falls prevention intervention.

Self-management
- Providing information about actions and behaviours that can prevent falls.
- Supporting the person living with a long-term neurological condition to identify behaviours that may increase the risk of falls.
- Signposting to local and national resources for advice and support.
- Providing advice and support on how to summon help should a fall occur.
- Promoting the use of telecare such as pendant alarms or remote monitoring, for example falls detector.
- Maximising individual capacity and control over life by encouraging health promoting behaviours.

7.7 Pain management

It is estimated that up to 75% of people living with a long-term neurological condition experience significant pain (Bragin et al., 2015). Pain alters physical and emotional functioning, decreases quality of life and impairs the ability to work (Ashburn and Staats, 1999). People living with a long-term neurological condition who develop chronic pain typically experience related depression, sleep disturbance, fatigue and decreased overall physical functioning (Ashburn and Staats, 1999). Management of chronic pain requires a comprehensive approach to rehabilitation provided in a co-ordinated manner (Ashburn and Staats, 1999) and can include medication including opioid analgesics, anti-depressants and behavioural approaches.

Occupational therapists can contribute through supporting the person living with a long-term neurological condition to change patterns of negative thoughts and attitudes to foster more healthy adaptive thoughts, emotions and actions (Ashburn and Staats, 1999). A pain management programme includes four key components: education, skills acquisition, cognitive and behavioural rehearsal, and generalisation and maintenance (Ashburn and Staats, 1999).

7.7.1 Practical strategies for pain management

The following practical strategies for pain management have been adapted from Wanlass and Fishman (2011).

Pacing

Often people living with a long-term neurological condition describe patterns of 'good' and 'bad' days. People generally mean how much their symptoms, in this case pain, get in the way of their daily activities. Some people try to take advantage of the 'good' days by using them as days to catch-up, doing all the things they could not do on days when their pain was overwhelming. The result of over-doing activities on a catch-up day means people may need several days of rest to recover. Effective pacing means the persons living with a long-term neurological condition are in charge of how they plan, start, stop and change what they are doing. With effective pacing some activities can be achieved every day. Practical examples of pacing include the following:

- Breaking tasks into smaller parts, taking rests in between tasks
- Working at a slower, less intense pace
- Gradually increasing the amount of time spent doing a specific task
- Changing tasks often and using different parts of the body throughout the day.

Leading a healthy lifestyle

Eating regular, nourishing, high-fibre meals and drinking plenty of fluids are important to healing, managing pain and staying well.

- Drinking plenty of water is the best way to stay hydrated and avoid constipation. It is best to limit carbonated drinks, tea or coffee.
- Regular healthy eating helps to maintain energy levels, manage constipation and manage pain. However it is important to remember that some medications are best taken with food. This can help decrease nausea and avoid other possible side effects.
- Alcohol may interact with medications and cause serious side effects. It may interfere with the ability to get deep, restful sleep and may make emotions harder to deal with.
- Smoking impairs healing and can interfere with the body's ability to manage pain.

Using medications properly

Some people find it helpful to have a medication plan. Knowing the names of medications, what they are for, how and when to take them, and potential harmful side effects can help the person living with a long-term neurological condition make an individual plan that works best for them. Suggestions for managing medication include the following:

- Keeping an updated file of all current medications that includes all the written instructions about your medications.
- Using a pill box or dosette with appropriate doses sorted out for each day and time the medication will be taken.

- Using a timer or mobile phone alarm to remind you when to take your medication.
- Depending upon when the medication should be taken, linking it to another routine daily activity such as eating a regular meal, brushing your teeth or preparing for bed.

Exercise

Participation in regular exercise can improve the body's strength, flexibility and endurance. There may be times when it is necessary to lower activity levels due to illness or to recover from an acute, painful injury. However, this is not typically recommended for managing chronic pain. Repeated use of rest and avoidance of movement to temporarily reduce pain can lead to a decrease in strength, flexibility and endurance, and an increase in disability. Strategies for increasing exercise include the following:

- Identifying the activities you enjoy most and are most likely to do
- Finding a local group/friend/family member who may also have an interest
- Considering how this can be incorporated into your daily/weekly/monthly schedule
- Starting exercise gently, do not overdo it
- Gradually building up level of activity and always be aware of your body's response to exercise
- Allowing sufficient time for rest between exercise.

Stress, tension and pain

Increases in stress and tension can worsen pain. Pain itself may also be a source of stress. This can feel like a vicious circle that is difficult to break. The tension experienced in response to stress can be emotional such as being worried, fearful or frustrated. Stress can also affect how the person living with a long-term neurological condition can think. Tense muscles, as a result of stress, can aggravate some forms of pain and can use up energy that might be required for other tasks. Restoring the body's energy requires adequate rest, relaxation and proper nutrition. Techniques such as controlled breathing, muscle relaxation and visual imagery can all help to reduce stress and subsequently reduce pain (see section on Anxiety management page 129 section 7.5).

Shifting focus

People living with a long-term neurological condition may find that many aspects of their life have been pushed aside because of their pain or have found that pain seems to occupy most of their thoughts and behaviours. Perceptions of pain change according to the level of focus. Participation in meaningful occupations can distract the mind away from pain. Participation in enjoyable activities can help reduce attention to pain and help the person living with a long-term neurological condition to rediscover ways to enjoy life.

Thinking constructively

The occupational therapist should take time to explore underlying pain beliefs and help the person living with a long-term neurological condition cope with pain in a more useful way. Common pain beliefs include the following:

- My pain makes it impossible to do anything constructive or enjoyable.
- It is primarily the responsibility of my doctor to relieve pain.
- It is best to avoid all painful activity so I do not cause more injury.
- My attitudes and emotions don't affect how much I suffer from pain.

Socialisation and recreation

Pain often leads to a reduction or disengagement from social and recreational activities. People living with a long-term neurological condition may feel that they cannot contribute socially as they did previously or that they cannot keep up with their friends and so they withdraw leading to social isolation. This can ultimately lead to low mood and a heightened focus on pain and disability. The occupational therapist can support the person living with a long-term neurological condition to find ways to maintain socialisation or to find new or alternative occupations which provide meaning and purpose.

Ergonomics

The goal of ergonomics is to design tasks, tools, furniture and equipment in a way that minimises risk of injury and improves efficiency. The principles of ergonomics can be applied in any setting. Examples of good ergonomics include the following:

- Moving items to lower shelves to reduce physical stress
- Using appropriate postures and movements
- Using assistive devices.

7.8 Managing tremor

Current rehabilitation strategies aimed at minimising tremor include medication, compensatory strategies and assistive devices. There is however a lack of evidence to support the use of these approaches and indeed clinical trials have indicated the side effects of drugs such as Propanolol and Isoniazid often prevent optimal use (Bozek et al., 1987; Koller, 1984).

Proximal stabilisation utilises techniques which offer support to the affected hand while engaging in meaningful activities. The hand-over-hand technique as illustrated in Figure 7.1 involves the person living with a long-term neurological condition placing the non-dominant hand firmly on top of the dominant hand providing additional support while carrying out a task. This self-discovery strategy can reduce frustration and enhance function with evidence of continued use once the technique has been developed (Hawes et al., 2010).

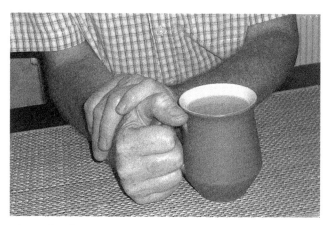

Figure 7.1 Hand-over-hand technique. (Source: Photographer and copyright J. Edmans 19.07.2015.)

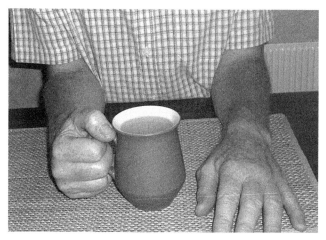

Figure 7.2 Distal stabilisation technique. (Source: Photographer and copyright J. Edmans 19.07.2015.)

Distal stabilisation incorporates strategies such as pressing the elbow firmly into the side of the trunk or resting the elbow on the table (see Figure 7.2). The key aim of distal stabilisation is to reduce the travelling distance, that is the distance the food travels from the plate to the mouth. Alternative methods might include lowering the head or bringing the entire torso toward the object (Hawes et al., 2010). People living with a long-term neurological condition and experiencing head tremor may attempt to stabilise the head against the shoulder in an attempt to reduce the tremor. Retracting the shoulder girdle and pressing it against the back of the chair or fixing the elbow in a locked straight position may give improved distal control (Multiple Sclerosis Trust, 2011). Provision of a head support attached to the chair may also provide distal support to help reduce head tremor.

Weighted cuffs can be applied to the distal upper extremity to decrease tremor in skilled movement (McGruder et al., 2003). The underlying belief is that weighted cuffs will be effective due to the proprioceptive input and fundamental biomechanical principles (McGruder et al., 2003). The amount of weight to be used however causes some controversy with estimates of weights between half and two pounds required to make a functional difference (Hawes et al., 2010). Weighted cuffs can be difficult to apply and cumbersome to wear and have in some circumstances been proven to decrease function or even make tremor worse (Hawes et al., 2010). Too much weight may also be worse than, or no better than, no weight at all (McGruder et al., 2003). Prolonged use of weighted cuffs should be avoided as the amplitude of the tremor can increase after the weights have been removed (Multiple Sclerosis Trust, 2011).

Cooling: Since the late 1950s, body cooling techniques have been applied to people with MS demonstrating improvement of several clinical symptoms including reduction in tremor (Meyer-Heim et al., 2007). Peripheral cooling does not impact on the core body temperature and is understood to reduce tremor amplitude and frequency by reducing the sensory input provided by muscle spindle afferents (Feys et al., 2005) although the main physiological mechanisms are not yet thoroughly understood (Meyer-Heim et al., 2007). Peripheral cooling for tremor requires the application of a cooling system to the forearm. Cooling systems operate through different mechanisms but generally involve circulation of a cooling liquid, air attached to a heat exchanger unit or vests with ice packs placed in pockets (Meyer-Heim et al., 2007).

Deep (18 °C) and moderate (25 °C) cooling interventions applied for up to 15 minutes reduced skin temperature at the elbow by 13.5 and 7 °C, respectively, with improved performance observed for up to 30 minutes after cooling (Feys et al., 2005). Peripheral cooling applied to the forearm has been proven to reduce overall tremor amplitude and frequency without compromising the accuracy of movement in people with MS (Feys et al., 2005).

Splinting can have variable results on tremor with some people finding minimal benefit, while others found it made tremor worse (Hawes et al., 2010). Made-to-measure Lycra garments are also being trialled to minimise tremor through sustained compression, stretch and proprioceptive feedback.

Assistive devices include low-tech devices such as weighted cutlery and pens through to assistive technology (see Chapter 8). In addition to altering the weight of utensils, it may be worth considering alternative grips as built-up, soft, comfortable pen grips may also assist in activities such as writing (Hawes et al., 2010). Electronic eating devices may also help some people living with a long-term neurological condition to maintain independence in an important aspect of occupational performance. Using mobile arm supports may also dampen tremor while supporting the upper limb and minimising fatigue.

7.9 Sleep

Within the context of the International Classification of Functioning, Disability and Health (World Health Organisation, 2002), sleep disorders can have a significant impact on a person's functioning at various levels, including body functions (i.e. energy, drive or attention), activities and participation (as in recreation and leisure or in carrying out daily routines), and environmental factors (i.e. preparing the environment for sleep, interactions with others who share the sleeping space and ensuring safety) (American Occupational Therapy Association, 2008; Gradinger et al., 2011).

> Occupational therapists use knowledge of sleep physiology, sleep disorders, and evidence-based sleep promotion practices to evaluate and address the functional implications of sleep insufficiency or sleep disorders on occupational performance and participation. (American Occupational Therapy Association, 2012)

Assessment of sleep should include (American Occupational Therapy Association, 2012) the following:
- Difficulties in sleep preparation
- Sleep participation
- Sleep latency (how long it takes to fall asleep, typically 30 minutes for someone without a sleep disorder)
- Sleep duration (the number of hours of sleep, which varies by age)
- Sleep maintenance (the ability to stay asleep)
- Daytime sleepiness
- The impact of work, life events, caregiving responsibilities
- The influence of pain and fatigue
- Disturbances in balance, vision, strength, skin integrity and sensory systems
- Psycho-emotional status, including depression, anxiety and stress
- The impact of caffeine, nicotine, drugs or alcohol, smoking or medication (e.g. prescriptions or over-the-counter sleep aids)
- The impact of the environment.

Occupational therapy interventions should focus on promoting optimal sleep performance and include (American Occupational Therapy Association, 2012) the following:
- Education on sleep terminology, misconceptions and expectations
- Preventing secondary conditions that may diminish sleep quality, for example decreased range of movement, depression or anxiety
- Encouraging smoking cessation, reduced caffeine intake, a balanced diet, adequate exercise
- Establishing predictable routines, including regular times for waking and sleeping
- Managing pain and fatigue
- Addressing activities of daily living, particularly for bed mobility and toileting

- Establishing individualised sleep hygiene routines (habits and patterns to facil-itate restorative sleep)
- Teaching cognitive-behavioural and cognitive restructuring techniques, such as leaving the bedroom if awake and returning only when sleepy, or exploring self-talk statements regarding sleep patterns
- Increasing coping skills, stress management, and time management
- Addressing sensory processing disorders and teaching self-management or caregiver management
- Modifying the environment, including noise, light, temperature, bedding and technology use while in bed
- Introducing complementary mind-body techniques, including progressive muscle relaxation, visual imagery, autogenic training, tai chi, yoga, meditation and biofeedback.

7.10 Sexual relationships and intimacy

While it is important to recognise that many people have sexual and relationship issues at some stage in their life, diagnosis with a long-term neurological condi-tion can have a significant impact on even the healthiest of relationships (Parkinson's UK, 2014; Table 7.1). Changes in mood and emotions including feelings of anger, frustration, denial or guilt may occur in response to the onset of disability and can impact upon communications, self-esteem and sexual desire (Parkinson's UK, 2014). As roles change different expectations may become apparent as one partner may wish to talk about the changes, while the other prefers to reflect on them alone (Parkinson's UK, 2014). Changing roles as couples move into the roles of 'carer' and 'cared for' can impact on perceptions of equality within a relationship. Physical intimacy is a crucial part of many relationships; however, some symptoms may make it more difficult to be spontaneous. Practical solutions within the home environment may also lead to couples sleeping in separate beds or even separate rooms.

The National Institute for Health and Care Excellence (NICE) clinical guideline (NICE, 2003) recognises the importance of enjoying sexual health regardless of illness and disability and states 'every person (or couple) should be asked sensi-tively about or given opportunity to remark upon, any difficulties they may be having in establishing sexual or personal relationships'. People do not always share their concerns, and occupational therapists are sometimes reluctant to enquire, but people with long-term neurological conditions should be offered the opportunity to discuss any issues or concerns (Multiple Sclerosis Trust, 2011).

7.10.1 General tips for improving relationships
The following general tips for improving relationships have been adapted from Parkinson's UK (2014).

Table 7.1 Types of sexual dysfunction and potential solutions.

Impairment	Sexual dysfunction	Potential solutions
Movement problems	• Stiffness • Rigidity • Slowness of movement • Involuntary movements • Spasticity • Pain	• Sexual positions may need to be altered to ensure the affected partner is stable and well supported
Fatigue	• Tiredness • Loss of desire	• Medication • Having intercourse at a different time of the day
Bowel problems	• Pain or tiredness • Low self-esteem • Vulnerability • Embarrassment and shame • Anger and resentment • Fear and anxiety • Guilt and self-blame • Depressed • Feeling dirty and unclean	• Enemas or laxatives before sexual intimacy • Anal plugs • Absorbent pads or underwear • Careful washing/showering prior to sexual contact
Bladder problems	• Urinary leakage during intercourse • Odour from leaking urine • Irritation to the genital area • Presence of drainage bag and/or catheter • Premature ejaculation • Vaginal dryness • Loss of sensation • Loss of desire for intercourse • Pain or tiredness • Low self-esteem • Vulnerability • Embarrassment and shame • Anger and resentment • Fear and anxiety • Guilt and self-blame • Depressed • Feeling dirty and unclean	• Careful washing/showering prior to sexual contact • Use geranium essential oil on adjacent clothing (not directly to skin!) • Empty the bladder just before any sexual activity • Put bed-protective sheets on the bed, have baby wipes and extra towels close by • Reduce fluid intake a few hours before sexual activity • Men could wear a condom if dribbling small amounts of urine • Sexual positions may need to be altered to minimise potential problems, for example remaining on your bottom if you fear you may leak on your partner • Males: tape catheter down the side of the penis and wear a condom • Females: tape catheter to abdomen (rear-entry position may be more practical). Catheter may be removed from bag and reconnected afterwards • Intermittent self-catheterisation can be done prior to intercourse
Erectile dysfunction	• Difficulty getting an erection • Getting an erection then losing it too soon	• Viagra/Cialis/Levitra • Self-injection • Pessary
Orgasm	• Absent orgasms • Premature ejaculation • Delayed ejaculation • Not ejaculating at all	• Minimise anxiety • Spend more time on general arousal and excitement • Masturbation • Sex aids

(continued)

Table 7.1 (Continued)

Impairment	Sexual dysfunction	Potential solutions
Hypersexuality	• Impulsive behaviour • Compulsive behaviour • Risk of socially unacceptable behaviour or breaking the law • Sexual delusions and hallucinations • Can be distressing for partner if sexual desires feel out of control and are out of character	• Behavioural interventions • Seek help from a psychosexual therapist
Female sexual dysfunction	• Loss of libido • Lack of vaginal lubrication • Difficulty in achieving orgasm • Pain during intercourse • Numbness	• Vaginal lubrication • Use of vibrators and sexual aids to increase the intensity of stimulation • Explore other means of achieving orgasm and additional erogenous zones • Find new ways to approach altered sexual functioning

Source: Based on Blackhouse et al. (2011), Multiple Sclerosis Trust (2011), Parkinson's UK (2014) and Huntington's Disease Association (2012).

- Love yourself: a strong relationship starts with positive self-esteem. If you don't love yourself, it is hard to believe anyone else will.
- Accept difference: we're all unique, so differences of opinion are a part of life. Accept arguments as a healthy part of life as a couple.
- Argue well: when you argue, make sure you confront the issue, not each other. Listen, be respectful and try to find a common solution.
- Say sorry: love does not mean never having to say you're sorry. We all make mistakes and can be wrong, so be ready to apologise.
- Listen and learn: people change and grow over time. Don't ever think you know your partner so well that you can predict what they're going to say.
- Make good quality time: make sure you make time to talk, laugh, chat or just be together.
- Share goals: talk about and work towards common goals.
- Spend time with other couples: it's easy to think that only you have problems, but when you spend time with other couples, you'll see you're not alone. All relationships have their ups and downs.
- Give each other the benefit of the doubt: don't jump to conclusions about each other's behaviour or motivation.

7.11   Self evaluation questions

1 What are the broad outcomes of rehabilitation?

2 What are the current rehabilitation strategies for managing tremor?

3 What are the general principles of cognitive rehabilitation?

4 What does 'generalisation' mean in relation to cognitive rehabilitation?

5 What are the key principles of fatigue management?

6 What are the symptoms of anxiety?

7 What are the strategies for managing pain?

8 What factors contribute to a good sleep?

9 What are the key interventions within falls management?

10 How can the occupational therapist support the client to maintain intimate relationships?

References

American Occupational Therapy Association (2008) Occupational therapy practice framework: domain and process, 2nd edition. American Journal of Occupational Therapy, 62:625–683.

American Occupational Therapy Association (2012) Fact sheet: occupational therapy's role in sleep. Bethesda, MD: American Occupational Therapy Association.

Aragon A and Kings J (2010) Occupational therapy for people with Parkinson's: best practice guidelines. London: College of Occupational Therapists and Parkinson's UK.

Ashburn MA and Staats PS (1999) Management of chronic pain. The Lancet, 353:1865–1869.

Blackhouse M, Wiley D, Wylie K and Allen P (2011) Sex and incontinence: information for patients. Sheffield: Sheffield Teaching Hospitals NHS Foundation Trust.

Bozek CB, Kastrukoff LF, Wright JM, Perry TL and Larsen TA (1987) A controlled trial of isoniazid therapy for action tremor in multiple sclerosis. Journal of Neurology, 234:36–39.

Bragin I, Dvoskin D, Zidan A, Joseph R and Thomas PS (2015) Characteristics of neurology referrals to pain management. Neurology, 84(14S):P3.309.

Brooks NA and Matson RR (1982) Social-psychological adjustment to multiple sclerosis: a longitudinal study. Social Science and Medicine, 16(24):2129–2135.

Busse M, Wiles CM and Rosser AE (2009) Mobility and falls in people with Huntington's disease. Journal of Neurology and Neurosurgery and Psychiatry, 80:88–90.

College of Occupational Therapists (2015) Occupational therapy in the prevention and management of falls in adults. Practice guideline. London: College of Occupational Therapists.

Cook C, Page K, Wagstaff A, Simpson S and Rae D (unpublished) Occupational therapy for people with Huntington's disease: best practice guidelines. Birmingham, UK: European Huntington's Disease Network.

Feys P, Helsen W, Liu X, Mooren D, Albrecht H, Nuttin B and Ketelaer P (2005) Effects of peripheral cooling on intention tremor in multiple sclerosis. Journal of Neurology, Neurosurgery and Psychiatry, 76(3):373–379.

Gradinger F, Glässel A, Bentley A and Stucki A (2011) Content comparison of 115 health status measures in sleep medicine using the ICF as a reference. Sleep Medicine Reviews, 15(1):33–40.

Gunn HJ, Newell P, Haas B, Marsden JF and Freeman JA (2013) Identification of risk factors for falls in multiple sclerosis: a systematic review and meta-analysis. Physical Therapy, 93:504–513.

Hagedorn R (2001) Foundations for practice in occupational therapy. Edinburgh: Churchill Livingstone.

Harrison S (2007) Fatigue management for people with multiple sclerosis, 2nd Edition. London: College of Occupational Therapists.

Hawes F, Billups C and Forwell S (2010) Interventions for upper-limb intention tremor in multiple sclerosis: a feasibility study. International Journal of MS Care, 12:122–132.

Huntington's Disease Association (2012) Sexual problems and HD. Liverpool: Huntington's Disease Association.

Koller K (1984) Pharmacologic trials in the treatment of cerebellar tremor. Archives of Neurology, 41:280–281.

McGruder J, Cors D, Tiernan AM and Tomlin G (2003) Weighted wrist cuffs for tremor reduction during eating in adults with static brain lesions. American Journal of Occupational Therapy, 57:507–516.

Meyer-Heim A, Rothmaier M, Weder M, Kool J, Schenk P and Kesselring J (2007) Advanced lightweight cooling-garment technology: functional improvements in thermosensitive patients with multiple sclerosis. Multiple Sclerosis, 13:232–237.

Moodjuice (2015) Anxiety moodjuice self-help guide. Falkirk, Scotland: Adult Psychological Services, NHS Forth Valley. Available at http://www.moodjuice.scot.nhs.uk/anxiety.asp (Accessed 2 May 15).

Multiple Sclerosis Trust (2011) Multiple sclerosis information for health and social care professionals, 4th Edition. Hertfordshire: Multiple Sclerosis Trust.

National Institute for Health and Clinical Excellence (NICE) (2003) Clinical guideline 8 multiple sclerosis – management of multiple sclerosis in primary and secondary care. London: National Institute for Health and Clinical Excellence.

Nilsagard Y, Lundholm C, Denison E and Gunnarsson LG (2009) Predicting accidental falls in people with multiple sclerosis: a longitudinal study. Clinical Rehabilitation, 23:259–269.

Parkinson's UK (2014) Intimate relationships and Parkinson's. London: Parkinson's UK.

Post-White J and Fitzgerald M (2002) Imagery. In Snyder M and Lindquist R (Eds) Alternative/complementary interventions: a guide for nurses, 2nd Edition. New York: Springer.

SANE (2015) Anxiety factsheet. London: SANE Mental Health Charity.

Senders A, Wahbeh H, Spain R and Shinto L (2012) Mind-body medicine for multiple sclerosis: a systematic review. Autoimmune Diseases, 2012:567324. doi:10.1155/2012/567324.

Stolze H, Klebe S, Zechlin C, Baecker C, Friege L and Deuschl G (2004) Falls in frequent neurological diseases: relevance, risk factors and aetiology. Journal of Neurology, 251:79–84.

Stuifbergen AK, Becker H, Perez F, Morison J, Kullberg V and Todd A (2012) A randomized controlled trial of a cognitive rehabilitation intervention for persons with multiple sclerosis. Clinical Rehabilitation, 26:882–893.

Thomas S, Thomas PW, Nock A, Slingsby V, Galvin K, Baker R, Moffat N and Hillier C (2010) Development and preliminary evaluation of a cognitive behavioural approach to fatigue management in people with multiple sclerosis. Patient Education and Counselling, 78:240–249.

Toglia JP, Goliz KM and Goverover Y (2009) Evaluation and intervention for cognitive perceptual impairments. In: Crepeau EB, Cohn ES and Schell BAB (Eds) Willard and Spackman's occupational therapy. Philadelphia, PA: Lippincott Williams & Wilkins, pp. 739–776.

Von Groote PM, Bickenbach JE and Gutenbrunner C (2011) The world report on disability – implications, perspectives and opportunities for physical and rehabilitation medicine (PRM). Journal of Rehabilitation Medicine, 43:869–875.

Wahbeh H, Siegward ME and Oken BS (2008) Mind-body interventions. Neurology, 70(24):2321–2328.

Wanlass R and Fishman D (2011) Pain self-management strategies. California: UC Davis Medical Center, Department of Physical Medicine and Rehabilitation.

Wilson BA (1987) Rehabilitation of memory. New York: The Guildford Press.

World Health Organisation (2002) Towards a common language for functioning, disability and health: ICF. Geneva: World Health Organisation.

World Health Organisation (2011) World health organisation, world bank. World report on disability. Geneva: World Health Organisation.

World Health Organisation (2012) Concept paper world health organisation guidelines on health-related rehabilitation (rehabilitation guidelines). Geneva: World Health Organisation.

Worthington A (2007) Rehabilitation of executive deficits: effective treatment of related disabilities. In: Halligan PW and Wade DT (Eds) Effectiveness of rehabilitation for cognitive deficits. Oxford: Oxford University Press, pp. 257–267.

CHAPTER 8

Using technology to support participation

8.1 Introduction

Within the conceptual models of occupational therapy there is recognition of the complex relationship between the person and the environment. Environmental influences can both support and inhibit participation. Occupational therapy aims to facilitate positive interaction with the environment whilst recognising factors which contribute to restricted participation. Technology plays a key part in all our lives and has significantly advanced the range of potential solutions. This chapter offers practical guidance in the use of technology to support participation for people living with long-term neurological conditions.

8.2 Environmental characteristics and occupational performance

Theoretical models of occupational therapy conceptualise occupational performance as the 'dynamic interaction of person, occupation, and environment' (Townsend and Polatajko, 2007). The context of the person and occupational performance are described within earlier chapters of this book. The focus of the environment incorporates both the physical attributes and the social influences including culture and attitudes and how this enables or inhibits occupational performance. Aspects of the social aspects of the environment are considered within Chapter 9, allowing a more specific focus on the built environment throughout this chapter.

Occupational Therapy and Neurological Conditions, First Edition. Edited by Jenny Preston and Judi Edmans.
© 2016 John Wiley & Sons, Ltd. Published 2016 by John Wiley & Sons, Ltd.

The World Health Organisation (WHO, 2002) defines environmental factors of the International Classification of Functioning, Disability and Health (ICF) within the following broad categories:

- Products and technology
- Natural environment and human-made changes to the environment (built environment)
- Support and relationships
- Attitudes
- Services, systems and policies.

The built environment is defined within the features and characteristics of the surroundings in which people living with long-term neurological conditions engage in meaningful occupations. This will differ for each individual depending on their roles and occupations. The ability to successfully interact with the environment is determined by individual attitude and skills and not at an impairment level such as low vision or difficulty bending (Stark et al., 2015). Understanding and describing the range of environmental factors that impact on occupational performance is difficult given the vast number of environments and different features associated with each (Stark et al., 2015).

Occupational therapists employ a range of strategies to facilitate positive interaction with the environment including the following (Stucki et al., 2007):

- Approaches which build on and strengthen the resources of the person living with a long-term neurological condition, for example splinting
- Approaches which provide a facilitating environment, for example housing adaptations
- Approaches which develop performance in the interaction with the environment, for example provision of a wheelchair
- Approaches that enable the person living with a long-term neurological condition in their interactions with the environment, for example environmental control systems.

8.3 Environmental adaptations

Environmental adaptations refer to strategies that modify the physical environment with the goal of supporting and enhancing everyday competencies of people experiencing physical or cognitive problems due to long-term neurological conditions (Gitlin, 2015). There are three basic forms of environmental adaptations as follows:

1 Assistive technology
2 Structural changes or home modifications
3 Material adjustments, for example removal of rugs, rearranging furniture, adjusting lighting, colour coding or labelling.

8.4 Assistive technology

Assistive technology (AT) includes 'any item, piece of equipment, or product system, whether acquired commercially off the shelf, modified, or customised, that is used to increase, maintain, or improve functional capabilities of individuals with disabilities' (US Government Printing Office, 2004). An assistive device can be attached to the home structure, for example wall-mounted grab-rail; applied to the person, for example a splint; or directly manipulated by a person, such as an electronic eating device (Gitlin, 2015). Assistive technology is also referred to as 'special equipment' or 'assistive devices' and reflects a wide range of equipment and device choices of varying complexity and costs (Gitlin, 2015). Assistive technology can support participation by compensating for loss of function or enhancing residual skills and is classified in many different ways according to function, availability and specification (Polgar, 2015).

8.5 Assistive devices

Person-centred assessment practice is fundamental to the correct provision of assistive devices. This should be within the context of maintaining or promoting independence and should balance risk with the need to maximise functional potential and avoid over-provision (Scottish Government, 2009). It is essential that there is an individual outcomes-focussed approach to the assessment with clear goals identified, agreed, recorded and reviewed, with the provision of equipment seen as a 'means to an end' rather than being 'an end in itself' (Scottish Government, 2009). Carers are also entitled to an assessment in their own right (Scottish Government, 2009). Where equipment provided will be used by carers, then the occupational therapist should complete a full assessment of need which encompasses an appropriate risk assessment.

Assistive devices can support a range of needs and facilitate interventions including the following:
- Daily living, for example shower chairs and stools, raised toilet seats, bathing equipment, raised toilet seats, teapot tippers and liquid-level indicators
- Telecare products, for example flood detectors, falls monitors, smoke detectors and movement sensors
- Ancillary equipment for people with sensory impairments, for example flashing doorbells, low vision optical aids, text-phones and assistive listening devices
- Wheelchairs
- Environmental control equipment
- Communication aids including augmentative and alternative communication (ACC). (Scottish Government, 2009)

The term 'standard equipment' refers to 'equipment that can be used to meet simple to non-complex needs and which does not need to be adapted for the person living with a long-term neurological condition, such as shower chairs, raised toilet seats, bathing equipment, flashing doorbells and standard wheel-chairs' (Scottish Government, 2009). 'Specialist equipment' may 'require a more extensive and specialised assessment and is bespoke, uniquely specified and sourced for an individual (e.g. communication equipment, specially designed seating or wheelchairs)' (Scottish Government, 2009).

8.5.1 Provision following assessment

On completion of the assessment, the statutory context for the actual provision of equipment to meet the health or social care needs of the person living with a long-term neurological condition is determined by various legislative policies and localised procedures (Social Care Institute for Excellence, 2013). Provision of equipment may be determined by budgetary constraints and local eligibility criteria. If the person living with a long-term neurological condition is deemed eligible for support, the equipment is usually provided on a loan basis through a local equipment store (Social Care Institute for Excellence, 2013).

In England and Wales, under the Voluntary Retail Model, people who meet local eligibility criteria are offered a prescription (following an assessment) for a particular piece of equipment which can be exchanged at any accredited retailer in the their area or elsewhere (Consumer Focus, 2010). The equipment belongs to the client who is likely to be responsible for its maintenance (Social Care Institute for Excellence, 2013). It is also possible for people living with a long-term neurological condition to self-fund by purchasing assistive devices from specialist shops, via the Internet and mail order and, increasingly from some generalist retailers and charities (Social Care Institute for Excellence, 2013).

Occupational therapists that assess and order assistive devices are responsible for demonstrating the correct use of equipment and satisfying themselves as part of the assessment process that the equipment meets the assessed needs and the individual and carer(s) are safe in its use (Scottish Government, 2009).

8.5.2 VAT exemption

VAT legislation provides some relief for people with disabilities. There is no blanket exemption from VAT, and it is intended to apply to goods purchased which are designed solely for their use as a consequence of the disability. The following goods may qualify for VAT relief (HM Revenue and Customs, 2014):
- Some medical and surgical appliances
- Certain adjustable beds, chair lifts, hoists, lifts and sanitary devices
- Emergency alarm call systems
- Auditory training aids
- Low vision aids
- Specifically designed, or adapted, vehicles and boats
- Other equipment and appliances designed solely for disabled people
- Parts and accessories
- Repair and maintenance of goods.

8.6 Housing adaptations

A suitable, well-adapted home can be the defining factor in enabling the person living with a long-term neurological condition to live well and improve their quality of life (Scottish Government, 2009). Interventions should always be person-centred, and the occupational therapist should begin the process by understanding the experiences of the person living with a long-term neurological condition and helping to identify an individualised solution rather than proposing standardised approaches (Scottish Government, 2009).The provision of adaptations can reduce risk and injury, enabling carers to work safely and effectively and may prevent unnecessary admission to hospital, (Scottish Government, 2009).

8.6.1 Minor adaptations

Minor Adaptations are 'relatively inexpensive and may be fitted relatively easily and quickly such as grab-rails, handrails, flashing doorbells and smoke alarm alerts' (College of Occupational Therapists, 2006). Minor adaptations can be classified within the categories outlined in Table 8.1 (College of Occupational Therapists, 2006).

Table 8.1 Minor adaptations included in the guide.

1. Visual impairment needs	Staircase applications
	External lighting
2. Hearing impairment needs	Flashing doorbells
	Smoke alarm alerts
3. Rails	Main entrance support rail
	Grab-rails
	Newel rails
	Handrails
	Stair handrails
4. Access	Internal door threshold ramps
	Improved access and widened pathway to main entrances
	Door entry intercom
5. Kitchens and bathrooms	Window opening equipment
	Kitchen lever taps
	Kitchen cupboard handles
	Bathroom lever taps
	W.C. lever flush handles
	Bathroom grab-rails
6. General needs	Door and wall protectors
	Alter heights of electric faceplates
7. Safety matters	Safety glass
8. Highways	Drop kerbs

Source: College of Occupational Therapists 2006, Table 2.1, p. 7. Reproduced with permission of College of Occupational Therapists.

8.6.2 Major adaptations

Major adaptations involve 'extensive structural alterations or other permanent changes to a house, but excluding work to extend a structure to create additional living accommodation, or work to create living accommodation in a separate building from the current living accommodation' (Scottish Government, 2009). Major adaptations include the following (Scottish Government, 2009):

• Installation of ramps and widening doorways
• Adapting or providing a room to make it safer for the person living with a neurological condition
• Provision of a stair lift
• Provision of a level access shower.

The role of the occupational therapist in the provision of environmental adaptations

Occupational therapists are responsible for the following (Home Adaptations Consortium, 2013):

• Identifying and assessing the needs of people living with long-term neurological conditions
• Making recommendations about solutions to the assessed needs
• Preparing specifications and making practical arrangements to put those recommendations into practice
• Advising or administrating the financial support available.

Principles of the assessment

The purpose of an adaptation is to modify the home environment in order to restore or enable independent living, privacy, confidence and dignity for individuals and their families (Home Adaptations Consortium, 2013).

The focus is therefore on identifying and implementing an individualised solution to enable a person living within a disabling home environment to use their home more effectively rather than on the physical adaptation itself. It is important to take cognisance of where both the individual and their family are in the process of coming to terms with the condition and its potential progress, whilst taking into account the need to 'future proof' the home to take account of the likely course of the condition (Home Adaptations Consortium, 2013).

The appropriateness and acceptability of the adaptation outcome should be measured by the extent to which it meets the needs identified by the person living with a long-term neurological condition sensitively, efficiently and cost-effectively (Home Adaptations Consortium, 2013). The assessment process should be delivered sensitively, it is important to balance the benefits of any proposed adaptation to the potential levels of upheaval and timescales involved with some types of adaptations with the stage of the disease (Home Adaptations Consortium, 2013).

Consideration should be given to expedite procedures and interim solutions where some measure of delay is inevitable (Home Adaptations Consortium, 2013). Where it is likely that the adaptation will provide benefit for a limited period of time, for example for someone living with motor neurone disease (MND), this should not be automatically regarded as a sufficient reason for delaying or withholding its provision (Scottish Government, 2009).

Good clinical practice involves the following (Scottish Government, 2009):

- Placing the person living with a long-term neurological condition and their carer(s) at the centre of provision
- Enabling choice and control for people living with long-term neurological conditions and their carer(s) as partners in the process of assessment and support planning
- Focusing all care and support on the improvement of outcomes for the person living with a long-term neurological condition and their carer(s)
- Promoting a consistent approach to the assessment for, and provision of adaptations
- Ensuring that people living with long-term neurological conditions and their carer(s) have access to up to date and relevant information on equipment and adaptations
- Promoting good practice and partnership working in relation to adaptation provision.

8.7 Seating and postural management

Throughout our everyday lives we continually interpret and respond to stimuli within the environment which allows us to adjust our position and movements in response. Information regarding orientation and movement of the head, body and limbs in space is conveyed through highly integrated visual and somatosensory systems which contribute to control of balance and equilibrium (Mew and Winnall, 2010).

8.7.1 The role of normal posture as a foundation for occupational performance

In order to be stable enough to resist the forces of gravity but flexible enough to allow successful execution of efficient movement, normal postural control works to:

- Build posture up against gravity
- Fix the orientation and position of body segments
- Provide a reference point from which movement can be undertaken
- Maintain a stable but adaptable posture in line with task demands. (Edwards, 2002; Massion, 1994)

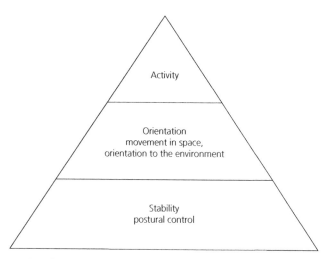

Figure 8.1 Hierarchy of normal postural ability. (Source: Harrison Training Manuals. Reproduced with permission of Harrison Training.)

When normal posture is compromised, balancing against the influence of gravity takes precedence over all other activities. This compromise can lead to stereotypical postures such as side flexion impacting on head position during eating or when attempting to communicate. Impaired balance mechanisms can also lead to the use of both lower and upper limbs to gain stability, severely limiting the use of upper limbs for occupational performance (Pope, 2007a; Raine et al., 2009).

Figure 8.1 illustrates a typical clinical reasoning hierarchy that occupational therapists should consider when supporting people living with progressive neurological disease to ensure optimum engagement with the environment. Bearing in mind the fluctuating and often unpredictable course of some neurological conditions, therapists should aim to achieve lower levels of the hierarchy before addressing higher levels in order to guarantee the safety and comfort of their clients.

People living with long-term neurological conditions who are unable to move through a full active range of movement, for example due to spasticity, rigidity, weakness or cognitive decline are vulnerable to developing contractures. A contracture is defined as the restriction of range of motion about a joint to such an extent that it causes limitations in activities of daily living, pain or skin breakdown. Research suggests that once established contracture is difficult and very time consuming to correct (Kilbride, 2015).

Eventually prolonged mechanical deformation of skeletal arrangement and/or immobility of joints and muscles can result in well-established intractable deformation of skeletal arrangement, for example scoliosis or hip and knee flexion contractures. Secondary complications due to biomechanical changes associated with immobility can be avoided if correct management strategies are used throughout a 24-hour period.

8.8 Management of posture and positioning in sitting

The main aim in sitting is to promote the correct posture and body alignment through the provision of adequate support. Figure 8.2 illustrates a step-by-step guide to building a stable seated posture.

8.8.1 Posture and head control in sitting

The impact of tonal changes can make maintaining an upright position against gravity difficult in sitting if suitable back, head and neck support is not available. The backrest of any form of seating must accommodate the shape of the spine; otherwise, head and neck control may be compromised (Rolfe, 2013). A forward flexed head can lead to the development of a kyphosis (Rolfe, 2013) and can contribute to difficulties with respiratory function, communication and swallowing.

There are a wide range of commercially available collars which can be considered; however, it is important to bear in mind that they have been designed

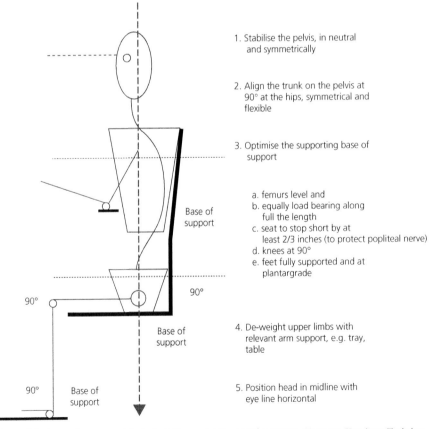

1. Stabilise the pelvis, in neutral and symmetrically

2. Align the trunk on the pelvis at 90° at the hips, symmetrical and flexible

3. Optimise the supporting base of support

   a. femurs level and
   b. equally load bearing along full the length
   c. seat to stop short by at least 2/3 inches (to protect popliteal nerve)
   d. knees at 90°
   e. feet fully supported and at plantargrade

4. De-weight upper limbs with relevant arm support, e.g. tray, table

5. Position head in midline with eye line horizontal

Figure 8.2 A step-by-step guide to building a stable seated posture. (Source: Harrison Training Manuals. Reproduced with permission of Harrison Training.)

primarily for immobilisation following neck trauma making them less suitable for people living with long-term neurological conditions (Alton et al., 2014). Immobilisation of the neck can make it difficult for people living with a long-term neurological condition to open their mouth, to be able to speak, eat and drink (Alton et al., 2014). Different types of collars may be required for different activities, for example the type of collar required for supporting the head while travelling in the car may be different to the type of collar used to support the neck during eating and drinking. Collars should be used in conjunction with other postural management equipment and techniques to ensure the correct combination for the person living with a long-term neurological condition (Alton et al., 2014).

Tilt-in-space chairs, wheelchairs or shower chairs, which include a mechanism that tilts the whole seat backwards, off-load the effects of gravity and provide support for the back and neck (Alton et al., 2014). Riser/recliner chairs with the tilt-in-space facility may provide appropriate postural support while reducing fatigue and improving general mobility (Rolfe, 2013). Riser/recliner chairs can also provide a safe and comfortable alternative to bed for people who tend to sleep during the daytime in addition to assisting people living with a long-term neurological condition who find it difficult to move from sitting to standing (Rolfe, 2013). The occupational therapist should however remain aware that by tilting equipment this may cause the person to become disoriented within their environment and may limit their communication (Huntington's Disease Association, 2012).

8.8.2 Wheelchairs

Making the decision to use a wheelchair can be quite significant for many people living with a long-term neurological condition with anecdotal evidence indicating that this can represent a key milestone in disease progression. The occupational therapist should however facilitate discussions in relation to occupational performance encouraging the person living with a long-term neurological condition to view the wheelchair as a mechanism for supporting engagement and participation. This may require a phased approach starting with the use of a manual wheelchair which can be stored within the boot of the car. The wheelchair can then be gradually introduced into the person's lifestyle as required. The use of practical examples of how the use of a wheelchair can support participation should be individualised by the occupational therapist who should also support the psychological adjustment to wheelchair use.

Manual wheelchairs are used to accommodate the needs of people who are beginning to experience mobility problems. Manual wheelchairs can be propelled by an attendant, or if there is sufficient upper limb movement and strength, by the person living with the long-term neurological condition. Manual wheelchairs can be adapted to provide more postural support as changes occur and when a powered wheelchair is neither wanted nor appropriate to clinical need (Rolfe, 2013). A highly supportive manual wheelchair will be larger than a standard wheelchair and will not fold easily into a car boot, especially if it includes a tilt-in-space mechanism (Eldridge et al., 2015).

8.8.3 Powered wheelchairs

Powered wheelchairs provide the person living with a long-term neurological condition with more independence for their own mobility if they are unable to self-propel a manual wheelchair (Eldridge et al., 2015). Powered wheelchairs can be operated by a range of input devices from a joystick controller to mouth controls. Assessment for a powered wheelchair is more complex and generally requires input from a wheelchair therapist or rehabilitation engineer (Eldridge et al., 2015).

Powered wheelchairs can be adapted to include tilt-in-space mechanism, riser function and additional postural support as the needs of the person living with a long-term neurological condition change. Statutory provision of powered wheelchairs will be determined by eligibility criteria and budgetary constraints and additional funding may be required for some adaptations. Powered chairs can be used for indoor/outdoor use although the additional weight of the wheelchair, motor and battery can make it difficult to lift a powered wheelchair into the boot of the car (Eldridge et al., 2015).

8.9 Management of posture and positioning in lying

Overnight positioning has become an increasing concern for occupational therapists as attempts to manage postural deficits during waking hours can be readily undone overnight (Goldsmith, 2000). Pillows and rolled-up towels can provide an effective means of increasing the individuals' acceptance of their base in lying and maintaining a more symmetrical alignment of body segments. The use of positioning aids such as electrically profiling beds, T-rolls and wedges can promote more equal loading of the tissues and improve alignment of body segments (Thornton and Kilbride, 2004).

8.9.1 Sleep systems

There are an increasing number of specially designed sleep systems on the market for clients who have very complex postural needs (Pope, 2007b). Sleep Systems are commercially available customised supportive mattresses which are used to maintain good posture when lying supine or on the side. Sleep systems however can be expensive to purchase, and it is recommended that a simpler means of night-time support such as the use of rolls and wedges is trialled before purchasing a more sophisticated system.

8.9.2 Bed mobility

People living with long-term neurological conditions may find that moving in bed becomes more difficult as their condition progresses. This can lead to increased risk of pressure sores particularly around the scapula and sacral areas. Loss of bed mobility can lead to feelings of discomfort and anxieties about being trapped, particularly if accompanied by impoverished or compromised respiratory function (Rolfe, 2013). Provision of bedrails can facilitate turning and rising from the bed although it is important to ensure that the rail is fitted at shoulder level of the bed occupant to provide a comfortable grip (Aragon and Kings, 2010).

Low-friction sheets and slide sheets can also help ease turning in bed. Some people may prefer to wear satin night-wear to support bed mobility, but this should not be used in conjunction with low-friction sheets as it may contribute to increased risk of sliding out of bed (Aragon and Kings, 2010).

8.9.3 Respiration

In many long-term neurological conditions, particularly MND, respiration may become impoverished as the condition progresses. The person living with a long-term condition will then require head support while lying in bed as they will no longer be able to lie flat. A mattress elevator or a profiling bed (see Figure 8.3) may be required to support the person to maintain this position. If non-invasive ventilation (NIV) is required, the person living with the long-term neurological condition will be required to sleep on their back with the head raised and the shoulders supported. Any equipment which is utilised should facilitate an elevated position from the hips and not the abdomen as this can further reduce respiration. Positioning to increase hip flexion will also assist to make the overall position more comfortable for the person living with a long-term neurological condition and where necessary will prevent sliding (Rolfe, 2013).

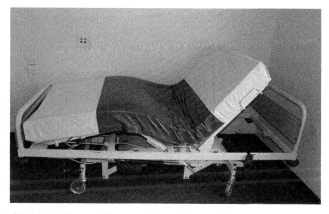

Figure 8.3 Profiling bed. (Source: Photographer and copyright J. Preston, 25.08.2015.)

8.10 Splinting

Splinting is an intervention used to support people living with a long-term neurological condition as part of a wider rehabilitation package. Splinting is used to maintain muscle length in the prevention and correction of contracture (Kilbride, 2015) and for improved comfort, pain relief, hygiene and sensory feedback. Splinting can also be used to improve function, for example typing, eating and writing.

8.10.1 Types of splints

There are two main types of splints: static and dynamic. Static splints are used to prevent movement, maintaining the forearm and hand in a functional position. Dynamic splints attempt to promote joint mobility and substitute absent muscle power through the use of controlled directional forces.

Splints can be custom-made from thermoplastic materials or purchased as off-the-shelf ready-made splints. The different types of splints have both advantages and disadvantages which need to be taken into consideration in the accurate assessment of the person living with a long-term neurological condition.

Key benefits of ready-made splints are that they are immediately available for use and do not rely on more specialist skills of the occupational therapist. Ready-made splints tend to be more comfortably padded and generally offer replacement covers to assist with hygiene.

Custom-made splints have the benefit of being made specifically to fit the individual and can be readjusted or remoulded as changes occur. However as it can take up to 2 hours to make a custom-made splint, it may not be possible for the person living with a long-term neurological condition to tolerate this due to problems such as fatigue. The occupational therapist is also required to have completed relevant training to ensure sufficient knowledge and skills in this area to avoid potential harm to the person living with a long-term neurological condition.

8.10.2 Assessing for a splint

A thorough, holistic assessment should be undertaken by the occupational therapist before deciding to recommend provision of a splint. Key factors of the assessment should include the following:

- Physical assessment of the upper limb including range of movement, sensation, muscle tone and skin care. Take account of factors such as posture and postural support, pain or possible infections. It is important to consider how the person living with a long-term neurological condition will be able to apply and remove the splint.
- Adherence to a clearly defined wearing schedule requires the ability to follow instructions and the ability to remember to apply or remove the splint. It is important to consider whether the person living with a long-term neurological

condition will be able to comply with this, that is motivation, memory and comprehension.

- Consideration should be given to wider environmental factors, for example is the person living with a long-term neurological condition able to get out of bed during the night to go to the toilet when the splint is applied?
- The overall goal of splinting should be clearly determined, for example increase range of movement, reduce pain and maintain ability to write. This should be determined by the person living with a long-term neurological condition in collaboration with the occupational therapist.
- If splinting is recommended, it is important to ensure that the occupational therapist has the necessary skills.

8.10.3 Education and monitoring

It is extremely important to educate the person living with a long-term neurological condition to ensure that the splint is worn correctly and therefore achieve the desired outcome. Where possible, written information (or alternative forms) should be provided which includes the following (College of Occupational Therapists, 2010):

- The purpose of the splint, including the advantages and the disadvantages
- When, and for how long the splint should be worn
- What exercises to do in conjunction with the splint
- How to apply and remove the splint
- How to determine if the splint is positioned correctly
- How to care for and clean the splint
- How to check the splint for pressure areas and swelling
- Contact details for the occupational therapist
- A review date.

8.11 Electronic assistive technology

Electronic assistive technologies (EATs) are integrated within everyday life with online shopping, instant messaging, digital photography and computer games becoming meaningful occupations for people living with long-term neurological conditions (Verdonck and Ryan, 2008). Mainstream technologies such as the Internet, computer software, computer hardware and portable devices including mobile phones, personal digital assistants (PDAs), personal organisers and alarms offer a range of functions that can be empowering for people living with long-term neurological conditions if considered fully by the occupational therapist (Verdonck and Ryan, 2008).

EAT is the umbrella term that describes electronic equipment that enables people with a physical disability to live more independently (Cook and Hussey, 2002; NHS England, 2013a). Occupational therapists have used EAT within their practice for many years, but there is a greater emphasis on the role of EAT with more recent innovations such as telehealth, telemedicine, smart housing and home automation (Verdonck et al., 2011).

High technology devices can be grouped together as EAT which is defined as 'a subset of assistive technology which comprises communication devices, environmental control systems, personal computers and the interface which permit their integration with information technology and with wheelchair control systems' (Royal College of Physicians, 2000). Occupational therapists are actively involved in the assessment and prescription, as well as the supply and maintenance of electronic assistive technologies (Verdonck et al., 2011). Yet challenges exist in maintaining a person-centred focus, limiting abandonment of technology and keeping up to date with emerging products while adhering to funding restrictions and organisational procedures (Cook and Polgar, 2008; Galvin and Donnell, 2002).

The benefits of EATs are reported to include positive perception of self-esteem, increased competence, increased adaptability and self-worth, decreased levels of frustration, decreased personal assistance time, improved quality of life, time alone and changed relationships (Verdonck et al., 2011). Electronic assistive devices can also support cognitive abilities by helping to manage daily lives, plan the day or week, remember appointments, keep contact information organised and keep track of notes (de Joode et al., 2010). People with cognitive deficits such as memory, planning, attention and motivational problems may also benefit from this type of support (de Joode et al., 2010).

8.11.1 Telehealth

Telehealth is defined as a service that 'uses equipment to monitor people's health in their own home…[monitoring] vital signs such as blood pressure, blood oxygen levels or weight' (Department of Health, 2009). People use the equipment within their own homes, and in some cases outside the home, to measure the vital signs that would normally be measured by a healthcare professional, helping to reduce frequent visits to the GP surgery. Telehealth is believed to contribute to a reduction in the number of unplanned hospital admissions by supporting self-management, particularly of long-term conditions. Data from the recording systems is transmitted automatically via broadband or a dial-up telephone line to a monitoring centre or healthcare professional. Readings that indicate changes outside the normal parameters which may indicate deterioration in health are then flagged for action (Davies and Newman, 2011). Telehealth might be used for people living with long-term neurological conditions to monitor respiratory function, cardiac function, blood pressure, blood sugar levels or weight.

8.11.2 Telecare

Telecare is defined as a service that uses 'a combination of alarms, sensors and other equipment to help people live independently. This is done by monitoring activity changes over time and will raise a call for help in emergency situations, such as a fall, fire or a flood' (Department of Health, 2009). Telecare therefore combines monitoring equipment with a monitoring service, and is most frequently used in the home. For those users with passive monitoring equipment, their behaviour patterns are monitored, and changes outside of their normal behavioural parameters are flagged for action (e.g. not getting out of bed at the usual time, exiting the house at night). This monitoring is intended to support people and enable them to continue living in their own home, independently or with the assistance of carers, for as long as possible (Davies and Newman, 2011).

8.11.3 Environmental control systems

Environmental control systems have been used for many years by people living with long-term neurological conditions to support them to live independently and perform activities within their own homes without assistance from others (Brandt et al., 2011). Through the use of an input device such as a switch or voice-controlled device, it is possible for people with physical impairment to control electronic equipment remotely, for example open and close doors and windows, utilise entertainment systems, telephones, alarms and computers with the aim of promoting autonomy and control of their lives (Brandt et al., 2011). Figure 8.4 provides a graphic representation of an environmental control system.

Possum Environmental Control System

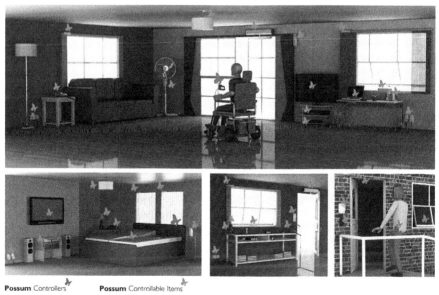

Possum Controllers   **Possum** Controllable Items

Figure 8.4 Illustration of an environmental control system. (Source: Possum Limited. Reproduced with permission of Possum Limited.)

8.11.4 Smart housing

More recent developments have seen the introduction of smart home technology which offers comparable but extended functionalities such as monitoring and automated functions, for example heating, roof windows automatically closing in the event of rain and lights automatically turning on when the person living with a long-term neurological condition gets out of bed (Brandt et al., 2011). A smart house is 'a house that has highly advanced automatic systems for lighting, temperature control, multi-media, security, window and door operations and many other functions' (Brandt et al., 2011).

8.11.5 Computer access

For many people living with a long-term neurological condition accessing a standard computer key board can become more challenging as their condition progresses due to impairments such as tremor, weakness, spasticity or altered sensation. Some inexpensive low tech solutions are available, for example a stylus, wrist supports and larger sized keys. Some standard operating systems such as Windows7® have an inbuilt accessibility feature which can alter the speed and pressure required to depress the keys which can be particularly helpful for people experiencing tremor. An onscreen keyboard can also be created for use in conjunction with a trackball mouse or head mouse.

Tablet devices may provide a lighter and easier means of accessing the Internet and other computer applications. Speech recognition software has become a standard application with Windows7® although external applications, for example Dragon Naturally Speaking® may provide a suitable alternative for some. Most speech recognition systems take time for the user to learn and require a consistency in speech production. This may not be a suitable option for people experiencing difficulties with dysarthria.

8.11.6 Switches and input devices

More specialist input devices may be required to operate computer systems, communication systems and environmental controls. A range of devices are available which allow control of the computer mouse by mouth piece, head control, foot pedal or switch or eye movements through the use of eye gaze control systems.

8.11.7 Augmentative and alternative communication

Augmentative and alternative communication include a range of methods of communication which can be used to add to the more usual methods of speech and writing when these are impaired and can be a way to help someone understand, as well as a means of expression (Scottish Government, 2009). This might include unaided systems such as signing and gesture (sometimes referred to as linguistic communication), as well as aided techniques ranging from picture charts to the most sophisticated computer technology currently available.

There are a range of computer programmes now available that can combine environmental control access with computer access and communication using eye gaze systems or switch control. This reduces the need for multiple input devices which can be tiring and difficult to manage. These can be programmed through a small tablet with a 10-inch screen which can be mounted on a wheelchair, or a larger monitor on a floor stand on wheels that can be positioned in front of a chair or over a bed. The occupational therapist should refer to the speech and language therapist for a more detailed specialist assessment for communication needs (NHS England, 2013b).

Case study: Beth

Person

Beth is 58 years old. She has been living with a diagnosis of multiple sclerosis (MS) for 24 years which has transitioned into secondary progressive MS within the past few years. Beth experiences muscle weakness in her upper limbs and she is unable to use her left (non-dominant) hand for any functional tasks. Beth has good head control but has some difficulty maintaining a symmetrical position when sitting on her chair. Beth has altered sensation which presents a risk regarding skincare. Beth has increased tone in her lower limbs, and she relies to some extent on this high tone in standing to transfer between her chair, bed, wheelchair and toilet. Beth experiences persistent visual impairment in the form of diplopia, intention tremor, and fatigue. Beth remains intact in her cognitive function and is able to make decisions about her own needs. Beth is very motivated to become more independent in her own home. She enjoys watching movies and listening to a wide range of music on the radio. Beth has many friends and enjoys keeping in touch with them through social media but has become low in mood as she is finding it increasingly difficult to use her computer.

Beth's occupational goals are as follows:

1 To operate the care line and have more flexibility over her care package
2 To be able to eat independently
3 To be able to sit more comfortably and feel more supported in her wheelchair
4 To manage her own finances by accessing digital banking services
5 To control the television independently
6 To control the radio independently.

Environment

Beth lives alone in a ground floor flat. She relies on a wheelchair to get around her home although she is not well supported in a self-propelled manual wheelchair. The effort involved in propelling the wheelchair is making Beth more fatigued, and this is leading to a further increase in tone. Currently Beth relies on the support of carers for all personal care. Beth has a level access shower facility in situ. Beth is currently using a static shower chair but is finding it increasingly difficult to transfer on and off this due to the increased tone in her lower limbs. Beth had previously fallen in the bathroom and has lost confidence transferring when the floor is wet.

Occupational therapy intervention

• Provision of joystick-controlled powered wheelchair with lateral supports in place to promote improved posture in sitting. Tilt-in-space function included but not currently required.

Pressure relieving cushion also provided. Extended footplate issued to provide additional support for feet.

- Electrically operated profiling bed provided to promote improved posture in lying and also to allow Beth to independently change her position during the night and further reduce the risk of damage to her skin.
- Wheeled shower chair with tilt-in-space facility issued. Beth can now be wheeled through to her bedroom to be dried fully and access the grab-rail in situ to allow additional support during her transfers.
- Beth was issued with an electronic eating device which dampens the tremor and allows her to eat independently. Beth is now enjoying a healthy and varied diet which is helping to promote her general health and well-being.
- Splint manufactured for night use for Beth's left hand to prevent contracture due to loss of function and mobility and to reduce pain.
- Provision of Possum 'Vivo' environmental control system with a large print menu set at a medium scan speed.
- Provision of joystick control to allow Beth to select the functions for operating the care line, telephone, television and radio. Beth can now control her environment and access the Internet for digital banking, social media and all other facilities this offers.

8.12   Self-evaluation questions

1 What are the four environmental factors within the ICF?
2 How can assistive technology support participation for people living with long-term neurological conditions?
3 What are the key differences between minor and major adaptations?
4 What factors impact on postural control?
5 What are the key stages to be considered when building a stable seated posture?
6 Why do contractures occur?
7 What is the difference between static and dynamic splinting?
8 How can electronic assistive devices assist a person with cognitive impairment?
9 How does telecare differ from telehealth?
10 What is an environmental control system?

References

Alton L, Broughton A, Knights C and Rolfe J (2014) Head supports for people with motor neurone disease. Northampton: Motor Neurone Disease Association.

Aragon A and Kings J (2010) Occupational therapy for people with Parkinson's: best practice guidelines. London: College of Occupational Therapists and Parkinson's UK.

Brandt A, Samuelsson K, Töytäri O and Salminen A (2011) Activity and participation, quality of life and user satisfaction outcomes of environmental control systems and smart home technology: a systematic review. Disability and Rehabilitation: Assistive Technology, 6(3): 189–206.

College of Occupational Therapists (2006) Minor adaptations without delay. Part 1: a practical guide for housing associations. London: College of Occupational Therapists.

College of Occupational Therapists (2010) Code of ethics and professional conduct. London: College of Occupational Therapists.

Consumer Focus (2010) Equipment for older and disabled people: an analysis of the market. London: Consumer Focus.

Cook AM and Hussey SM (2002) Assistive technology principles and practice, 2nd Edition. St Louis, MO: Mosby Publishers.

Cook AM and Polgar J (2008) Cook and Hussey's principles of assistive technology, 3rd Edition. St Louis, MO: Elsevier.

Davies A and Newman A (2011) Evaluating telecare and telehealth interventions. London: The Kings Fund.

Department of Health (2009) Whole system demonstrators: an overview of telecare and telehealth. London: Department of Health.

Edwards S (2002) Neurological physiotherapy: a problem solving approach, 2nd Edition. London: Churchill Livingstone.

Eldridge F, Jarvis K, Orr C and Rolfe J (2015) Wheelchairs for people with motor neurone disease. Northampton: Motor Neurone Disease Association.

Galvin J and Donnell C (2002) Educating the consumer and caretaker on assistive technology. In Scherrer MJ (Ed.) Assistive technology: matching device and consumer for successful rehabilitation. Washington, DC: American Psychological Association, pp. 325.

Gitlin L (2015) Environmental adaptations for individuals with functional difficulties and their families in the home and community. In Söderback I (Ed.) International handbook of occupational therapy interventions. Switzerland: Springer International Publishing, pp. 165–175.

Goldsmith S (2000) Postural care at night within a community setting. Physiotherapy, 86(10): 528–534.

HM Revenue and Customs (2014) VAT notice 701/7: VAT reliefs for disabled and older people. London: HM Revenue and Customs.

Home Adaptations Consortium (2013) Home adaptations for disabled people: a detailed guide to related legislation, guidance and good practice. Nottingham: Care and Repair England.

Huntington's Disease Association (2012) Seating, equipment and adaptations. Liverpool: Huntington's Disease Association.

de Joode E, Van Heugten C, Verhey F and van Boxtel M (2010) Efficacy and usability of assistive technology for patients with cognitive deficits: a systematic review. Clinical Rehabilitation, 24(8):701–714.

Kilbride C (2015) Splinting for the prevention and correction of contractures in adults with neurological dysfunction: practice guideline for occupational therapists and physiotherapists London: College of Occupational Therapists.

Massion J (1994) Postural control system. Current Opinion in Neurobiology, 4:877–887.

Mew M and Winnall S (2010) Management of visual and sensory impairments. In Edmans J (Ed.) Occupational therapy and stroke, 2nd Edition. Chichester: Wiley-Blackwell.

NHS England (2013a) Service specification complex disability equipment–environmental controls. Redditch: NHS England.

NHS England (2013b) Service specification complex disability equipment – specialised AAC services. Redditch: NHS England.

Polgar J (2015) Environment factors: technology. In Christiansen C, Baum C and Bass J (Eds) Occupational therapy: performance, participation and well-being, 4th Edition. Thorofare, NJ: Slack Incorporated, pp. 441–464.

Pope P (2007a) Severe and complex neurological disability: management of the physical condition. London: Elseveir.

Pope P (2007b) Night-time postural support for people with multiple sclerosis. Way Ahead, 11(4):6–8.

Raine S, Meadows L and Lynch-Ellerington M (2009) Bobath concept: theory and clinical practice in neurological rehabilitation. Chichester: Wiley-Blackwell.

Rolfe J (2013) Postural management in motor neurone disease: a guide to help maximise comfort and function in sitting and lying. Oxford: Oxford Motor Neurone Disease Care and Research Centre.

Royal College of Physicians (2000). Electronic assistive technology: a working party report of the British Society of Rehabilitation Medicine. London: Royal College of Physicians.

Scottish Government (2009) Guidance on the provision of equipment and adaptations. Edinburgh: Scottish Government.

Social Care Institute for Excellence (2013) Fair access to care services (FACS): prioritising eligibility for care and support. London: Social Care Institute for Excellence.

Stark S, Sanford J and Keglovits M (2015) Environment factors: physical and natural environment. In Christiansen C, Baum C and Bass J (Eds) Occupational therapy: performance, participation and well-being, 4th Edition. Thorofare, NJ: Slack Incorporated, pp. 387–420.

Stucki G, Cieza A and Melvin J (2007) The international classification of functioning, disability and health: a unifying model for the conceptual description of the rehabilitation strategy. Journal of Rehabilitation Medicine, 39:279–285.

Thornton H and Kilbride C (2004) Physical management of abnormal tone and movement. In Stokes M (Ed.) Physical management in neurological rehabilitation, 2nd Edition. Edinburgh: Elsevier, pp. 431–450.

Townsend E and Polatajko HJ (2007) Enabling occupation II: advancing an occupational therapy vision for health, well-being and justice. Ottawa, ON: CAOT Publications ACE.

US Government Printing Office (2004) 108th Congress. Assistive Technology Act of 1998, as amended, PL 108–364, PL 108–364, Section 3, 118 stat 1707. Washington, DC: US Government Printing Office. Amended October 25, 2004.

Verdonck M and Ryan S (2008) Mainstream technology as an occupational therapy tool: technophobe or technogeek? British Journal of Occupational Therapy, 71(6):253–256.

Verdonck M, McCormack C and Chard G (2011) Irish occupational therapist's views of electronic assistive technology. British Journal of Occupational Therapy, 74(4):185–190.

World Health Organisation (2002) Towards a common language for functioning, disability and health: ICF. Geneva: World Health Organisation.

CHAPTER 9

Living with a long-term neurological condition

9.1 Introduction

Throughout our lives we encounter a range of situations which require us to change or adapt as we move from one life phase to another. This process of adjustment can be easier for some than others and is believed to be dependent on a number of factors. This chapter will access theories of transitions in an attempt to understand the processes of adjustment and why some people living with neurological illness adapt more successfully than others. This will be placed within the context of occupational therapy practice and will consider the role of the occupational therapist in facilitating positive change.

9.2 Transitions theory

Transition refers to 'changes in our status that are discrete and bounded in duration although their consequences may be long-term' (George, 1993). Transitions are both a result of and result in changes in our lives, health, relationships and environments (Meleis et al., 2000). Successful transition is dependent on expectations, level of knowledge and skills, availability of new knowledge, available resources, capacity to plan for change and emotional and physical well-being (Schumacher and Mcleis, 1994).

Transition can be framed within four categories (Adams et al., 1976) as follows:
- Predictable – voluntary, for example most relationships
- Predictable – involuntary, for example national service
- Unpredictable – voluntary, for example blind date
- Unpredictable – involuntary, for example unexpected events such as diagnosis with a long-term neurological condition.

Occupational Therapy and Neurological Conditions, First Edition. Edited by Jenny Preston and Judi Edmans.
© 2016 John Wiley & Sons, Ltd. Published 2016 by John Wiley & Sons, Ltd.

Central to transitions theory is the concept of reconstruction of a valued self-identity (Kralik et al., 2006). Diagnosis with a long-term neurological condition can have a substantial cost to personal identity as people withdraw from former roles or perceive themselves to be failing within their existing roles, leading to a loss of self-worth and self-esteem (Preston et al., 2014). The importance of relationships and connections are also seen to be an integral part of successful transition (Kralik et al., 2006).

The types of transitions which may increase vulnerability for people living with a long-term neurological condition can be considered within three main categories as follows:

1 Illness experiences (e.g. diagnosis, surgical procedures, rehabilitation and recovery)
2 Developmental and lifespan transitions (e.g. pregnancy, childbirth, parenthood, adolescence, menopause, ageing and death)
3 Social and cultural transitions (e.g. migration, retirement and family caregiving) (Meleis et al., 2000).

9.3 Illness experiences

9.3.1 Diagnosis with a long-term neurological condition

The process of diagnosis with a long-term neurological condition can be challenging and lengthy given the lack of definitive diagnostic tests available. Receiving a diagnosis is usually a memorable and monumentous event accompanied by feelings of vulnerability and at times relief as people try to understand the meanings and consequences that the diagnosis holds for their present and their future (Kralik et al., 2001). Significant differences will be apparent within the diagnostic journey and the subsequent expectations for people diagnosed with a long-term neurological condition. Some people may receive the diagnosis with a resultant shock, anger and depression. For many this may immediately create a negative perception of life dependent on assistance from others or even premature death (Preston, 2009). For others who may have had previous experience of the condition, particularly in a hereditary condition like Huntington's disease (HD), their personal reflections may be drawn to the challenges of caring and the perceived burden of care on others.

Issues of fear, anxiety and uncertainty may be apparent not only at the diagnostic phase but also for some will continue throughout the course of their disease. Richard, diagnosed with multiple sclerosis (MS) nearly 40 years ago still reflects his anxieties as he describes how the disease has insidiously gnawed away at his life:

> I did a lot of reading on what it [MS] was, and eh…so I began to understand what it was wrong with me but then I started to get attacks, …my hands start…well I've always had my hands tingling, you know, that was the first thing, but gradually…other aspects crept

into my condition, it seems you get one condition and that diminishes and then before you know it another part of the condition occurs and just gradually over the years I mean…had, I lost the eyesight in my left eye, …I lost balance, then I was completely numb down one side of the body…um, so it just gradually built up with time and I had to decide how to get over these things. I mean at one stage when I had to get carried up the stairs, my kids and wife carried me up the stairs, well not carried me, pushed me up the stairs because I couldn't get up the stairs, well not on my own because I was completely paralysed down one side. That lasted about a month, and then it disappeared. As I say it creeps up on you and before you know it, bang it's there and you've got to deal with it some way. (Preston, 2009)

Lack of information at the time of diagnosis also impacted on the understanding and the subsequent perceptions of control for people living a life with MS. Jennifer recalls how reassured she felt when she was advised that she could have 20 years without any further incidents. Despite her initially positive expectations of a life with MS, her hopes were quickly dashed however when she experienced her first relapse after 2 years:

So my GP told me I could go another 20 years without another attack and I only lasted 2 years (laughs). And it just seems to get worse and worse with every attack. (Preston, 2009)

9.4 Rehabilitation and recovery

Rehabilitation within the context of long-term neurological conditions involves (Gutenbrunner et al., 2011):
1 Assessing functioning in relation to health condition, personal and environmental factors
2 Delivering interventions to:
  • Stabilise, improve or restore impaired body functions and structures
  • Prevent impairments and medical complications
  • Manage risk
  • Compensate for the absence or loss of body functions and structures.
3 Delivering programmes of intervention to optimise activity and participation through:
  • A person-centred problem-solving process
  • Working in partnership with the person with the long-term neurological condition
  • Working within a biopsychosocial framework
  • Applying and integrating biomedical and technological interventions
  • Education and counselling
  • Occupational, vocational and social support
  • Physical and environmental adaptations.

Occupational therapists have a key role to play in supporting people newly diagnosed with a long-term neurological condition as Paterson (2001) acknowledged the paradox of managing a condition which at times may be absent of symptoms but which requires acknowledgement of the limitations it creates on everyday life.

Early occupational therapy intervention should:

- Use open and genuine communication to encourage people newly diagnosed with a long-term neurological condition to tell their story and facilitate their coming to terms with the diagnosis
- Support people recently diagnosed with a long-term neurological condition to validate their experience by helping them to understand their symptoms and how they impact on their everyday lives
- Support the person living with a long-term neurological condition to find strategies which help them to cope with unpredictability and gain control of their lives
- Support the person living with a long-term neurological condition to mediate the effects of the disease through focussing on the emotional, spiritual and social aspects of life rather than primarily on the disease (Paterson, 2001).

9.5 Lifespan transitions

9.5.1 Parenthood

The decision to start a family should never be one that is taken lightly; however, additional factors may be required to be taken into consideration when you have been diagnosed with a long-term neurological condition.

Where there is a family history of a long-term neurological condition, for example HD or MND, there may be concerns about the risk that children will develop the condition in later life. For some this risk may feel too high, and they would rather avoid having children. Some couples may wish to consider gamete donation or adoption. Couples at risk to HD may find it more difficult to adopt although they may be able to undertake fostering. In vitro fertilisation (IVF) and artificial insemination by donation (AID) may also be considered (Huntington's Disease Association, 2012).

People living with a long-term neurological condition often worry about the practical aspects of parenting and how they will manage to look after their children. For Diana however there were different considerations as she reflected on a very poignant decision about her role of becoming a mother:

> Children. That was part of the marriage break up. I was, I was going for IVF, I was diagnosed with the MS...and that was okay. I went you know, went for the first month's course and...some woman that was in as well, she said 'do you think it is right for you to be doing IVF if you've got MS?' I said 'what do you mean?' So she said 'well, she says maybe you are going to have a child that will end up looking after you' so I thought, no I said because I wouldn't do that. So that was end of conversation. In the drive back home I thought about it and pulled over and I thought she's bloody right, I don't want to bring a life into this world that would maybe have to, well like at the moment

I couldn't carry the coffees through for my friends, they have to go and bring the coffees through themselves. So…you see children on the Red Nose day, there was that little girl looking after both her parents, mother and father, she was only 12, 13 and I thought… where's her childhood, she's not getting any, she's doing the dinner and she's doing the washing, she's doing the ironing and that broke my heart because I thought she's a baby. She needs to be having…fun with young friends, but…not doing things like that, but I don't, yeah…it's hard, don't get me wrong, it is hard but…I think it would be harder for me if I had them. How would I cope with this little life having to do this, that and the other for me and no…no…. (Preston, 2009)

The occupational therapist can support people living with a long-term neurological condition by:

- Providing information and support to help the person living with a long-term neurological condition to make informed decisions
- Supporting difficult decisions through the provision of emotional and psychological support
- Providing practical solutions to aspects of looking after a child, for example techniques for safe handling of a baby or small child; manipulating small fastenings when dressing a small child; or practical aspects to consider when choosing a pram or pushchair
- Providing strategies for fatigue management
- Environmental adaptation
- Developing strategies to compensate for loss, for example loss of mobility, loss of strength and cognitive changes

9.6 Social and cultural transitions

9.6.1 Work

Many people living with a long-term neurological condition are of working age at the time of symptom onset (Playford et al., 2011). Work is integral to daily life, providing financial support, emotional and psychological well-being, self-esteem, security and independence (Baldwin and Brusco, 2011). Maintaining work roles is therefore often a high priority for people living with a long-term neurological condition (Playford et al., 2011; Radford et al., 2013; Sinclair et al., 2014). Occupational therapists support people living with a long-term neurological condition to enter or return to work, remain in existing jobs, prepare and retrain for alternative job options and access appropriate alternative occupational and educational opportunities.

Vocational rehabilitation is 'a multi-professional evidence-based approach that is provided in different settings, services, and activities to working age individuals with health-related impairments, limitations, or restrictions with work functioning, and whose primary aim is to optimize work participation' (Escorpizo et al., 2011). Disability and return to work following diagnosis with a long-term neurological condition has been recognised as a process influenced by a variety of social, psychological and economic factors (Franche and Krause, 2002). Characteristics of the work environment, the health status of the individual and the insurance system all have a significant influence on return-to-work outcomes independent of the underlying medical condition (Franche and Krause, 2002).

Vocational rehabilitation is a process of engaging or re-engaging a person with work (Escorpizo et al., 2011). Return to work has been conceptualised as a continuum of events from being 'off work', 're-entry', 'retention' and 'advancement' (Young et al., 2005). Vocational rehabilitation is designed to maximise work participation of people living with a long-term neurological condition and to promote their full participation in society (Parker et al., 2005). Vocational rehabilitation involves the processes by which services improve a person's capacity for work, help them return to work or assume work duties at a permanent and sustainable level (Escorpizo et al., 2011).

Remaining in work

People living with a long-term neurological condition are less likely to remain in work when compared to those living with chronic diseases such as arthritis, diabetes or depression (Varekamp et al., 2008). Although more than 90% of people living with MS are employed prior to developing the disease, it is estimated that between 70 and 80% will become unemployed within 5 years of diagnosis (Strober et al., 2012).

Demographic aspects such as age, gender and level of education and disease-specific factors such as disease duration, disease course, neurological disability and symptomatic impairment have been found to be associated with employment status (Krause et al., 2013). Risk factors for unemployment among people living with long-term neurological conditions include female gender, low education level, high degree of neurological impairment and a progressive disease course (Strober et al., 2012). Males and older persons are more likely to leave work however because of a long-term neurological condition (Simmons et al., 2010).

Key factors which impact on the ability to remain in work include transport to and from work; moving around at work; equipment use; and impact of symptoms including fatigue, cognition balance and bladder dysfunction (Simmons et al., 2010). Once out of work the challenges of everyday job-hunting may be amplified for people living with long-term neurological conditions as they may need to overcome additional factors such as reduced confidence following a dismissal process, loss of benefits, gaps in their curriculum vitae (CV) and an uncertainty about if or when to disclose their diagnosis.

Disclosing a long-term neurological condition

People living with a long-term neurological condition are not legally required to disclose a health condition unless they work within the armed forces, onboard an aircraft or if their condition puts themselves or others at risk (HMSO, 2010).

Employers are not permitted to ask about health status or disability. The onus is on the person living with a long-term neurological condition to be honest as provision of false information could affect their employment at a later stage.

Early disclosure appears to support earlier adjustments being put in place for the person living with the long-term neurological condition. There can however be a strong fear that disclosure will result in discrimination resulting in loss of promotion or being sacked (Sweetland et al., 2007). Personal identity and trust may also be impacted by disclosure (Dyck and Jongbloed, 2000). Although employers will be concerned about the ability of the person living with a long-term neurological condition to meet the job requirements the evidence suggests that most employers want to do the right thing by valued employees and an appropriately timed and supported disclosure could well lead to a better understanding and more effective accommodation within the workplace (Simmons et al., 2010).

Occupational therapists can support disclosure by (adapted from Multiple Sclerosis [MS] Society, 2010):

- Providing advice and information on the individuals rights under the Equality Act (HMSO, 2010)
- Encouraging the person living with a long-term neurological condition to consider the pros and cons of disclosure specific to their industry, relationships at work, diagnosis and needs in the work place.
- Encouraging the person living with a long-term neurological condition to make a list of who they will disclose to, when, where and what information about their diagnosis and symptoms they are happy to share.
- Encouraging the person living with a long-term neurological condition to write a script of that they will say.
- Practice saying this out loud to others first as this can sometimes be an emotional experience.
- Positively frame the situation for example, 'Yes relapsing and remitting MS is unpredictable and I may not know when I may have a relapse, this could be in a few months' time but could also be in several years', 'I have a good medical care team who can help me manage my condition'.
- Encouraging the person living with a long-term neurological condition to make sure that any agreed adjustments are formally documented through Human Resource departments as future changes in management could affect these.

Equality Act

The Equality Act (HMSO, 2010) provides the legal statute to protect people living with disabilities from being disadvantaged in work. It stipulates that employers have a duty to make reasonable adjustments to the work place or working arrangements. However, what is considered 'reasonable' for the employer to implement is influenced by a number of factors such as how effective the change will be and its practicality, the cost of implementation and the size of the organization.

The Equality Act (HMSO, 2010) defines 'disabled' as a 'substantial' physical or mental impairment lasting longer than 12 months and that has a negative effect of the ability to carry out everyday activities of daily living.

Practical application of 'reasonable adjustment'

Hannah is 32 years old and has been employed within a large government organisation for the past 5 years as an administrator. Hannah was diagnosed with MS 10 years ago and in the last 12 months has been advised that this is a relapsing remitting form of the disease.

Hannah works 34 hours over a 4-day week. She lives in her privately owned house with two large dogs. She has paid support for dog walking but describes feeling guilty that they are indoors for most of the day, so she tries to make up for this at weekends by taking them for long walks. As a result she reports little energy for socialising at weekends and feels that she has lost contact with many of her friends.

Work difficulties identified

- Fatigue, exacerbated by long working days and impacts on all activities of daily living
- Difficulty writing and typing at speed, difficulty taking minutes or notes due to decreased coordination and tremor in her right hand
- Anxiety when under work pressure due to concerns about making mistakes
- Difficulties with concentration and remembering information especially when fatigued or anxious
- Right shoulder pain when typing and using a mouse.

Suggested adjustments

- Four-week trial of a change in working pattern from 4 long days to 3 long days and 2 half days; use of a Dictaphone during meetings where she is required to take minutes
- Use of Access to Work taxi to support with travel to and from work
- Ergonomic assessment of her work station
- Technological assessment and provision of voice activated software to aid typing fatigue and efficiency
- Relocation of desk to a quieter area of the office to aid concentration during focused periods of work.

Return to work

In most cases people living with long-term neurological conditions choose to leave their employment voluntarily and often before their illness has rendered them incapable of working (Rumrill et al., 2008). However, there is increasing evidence that people living with long-term neurological conditions may leave work prematurely. As many as 80% of people living with a long-term neurological condition who have voluntarily given up work believe they still have the ability to work and indicate that they would like to re-enter the workforce (Rumrill, 2009). People who receive disability benefits face particular difficulties in restarting their careers (Rumrill, 2009). It is therefore essential that people living with long-term neurological conditions are supported to make the correct decisions, at the right time, about their employment choices.

Early intervention is critical in supporting people living with a long-term neurological condition to reduce or remove job-related barriers before they undermine job satisfaction and, eventually threaten job retention (Roessler, 1996; Roessler and Rumrill, 1995). People living with a long-term neurological condition need to be able to re-access services as and when required. Consequently services should be open access and empower the person to take control of and manage their own situation (Roessler, 1996; Roessler et al., 2001, 2004).

Occupational therapists can support vocational rehabilitation approaches which include the following:
- Supporting people living with long-term neurological conditions with emotional self-management and support with disclosure and issues around discrimination.
- Empowering people living with long-term neurological conditions through education and support.
- Delivering interventions that focus on self-confidence and self-efficacy with regard to work-related problems.
- Supporting people living with long-term neurological conditions with work planning, effective decision-making, defining and implementing accommodations.
- Visiting the worksite to make more accurate assessment of need.
- Providing education about relevant legislation and how it applies to the person living with a long-term neurological condition, the nature of reasonable accommodation and advice on how to document any discrimination.
- Providing interventions that improve performance, compensate for changing performance or modify performance by reducing the demands of the task (Sweetland et al., 2007; Yorkston et al., 2003).
- Ensuring that strategies do not focus on reducing the Impairment but on performance of an activity (Sweetland et al., 2007; Yorkston et al., 2003).
- Minimising the impact of symptoms on work (Johnson et al., 2004).

Supporting employers
Employers play a key role in providing holistic and integrated care for people living with long-term neurological conditions to remain in work (Zheltoukhova, 2011).

Occupational Therapists can support employers by (Zheltoukhova, 2011):
- Providing accurate and relevant information about the neurological condition
- Providing a key resource to discuss aspects of the neurological condition and the potential impact of symptoms on the individual's performance at work

- Supporting employers to find practical realistic solutions within the workplace
- Enabling employers to provide a flexible working environment, including work schedules
- Providing information regarding schemes such as Access to Work as early as possible to support the employee living with a long-term neurological condition
- Working with GPs to support phased return to work according to the fit note
- Preserving job quality, avoiding excessive or damaging job demands and take heed of good ergonomic practice
- Providing tailored vocational rehabilitation to support return to work, productivity, morale and sustainability of performance.

9.6.2 Driving

Driving is a key part of life for many people living with a long-term neurological condition. Driving is an occupation in itself which provides meaning and purpose as people engage in driving for a number of reasons. There is general acceptance that driving promotes community mobility, supports maintenance of social networks and forms part of daily routines, for example taking children to school (Canadian Association of Occupational Therapists [CAOT], 2009). For others, driving promotes a sense of freedom and enjoyment. Consequently stopping driving is associated with lost social activities and depression even when other forms of transport are available (Hawley, 2001).

Common symptoms that may affect driving include the following:
- Sensory problems such as numbness or tingling in the hands and feet
- Visual problems such as blurred or double vision, temporary loss of visual, for example optic neuritis
- Fatigue
- Loss of muscle strength and dexterity
- Problems with balance and coordination
- Muscle stiffness and spasms including tightening or rigidity
- Difficulty with memory, concentration, spatial awareness, speed of processing
- Medications.

The role of the occupational therapist in relation to driving includes the following:
- Providing information about the law and driving with a long-term neurological condition
- Providing information about a person's fitness to drive
- Identifying the need for referral to a driving assessment centre for comprehensive assessment of driving ability
- Driver rehabilitation
- Providing information about vehicle modification
- Supporting driving cessation.

Driving and the Law

All drivers are legally responsible for informing the Driver and Vehicle Licensing Agency (DVLA) following diagnosis with MS, MND, HD or Parkinson's. However not all drivers notify the DVLA when there is cause for concern. For some it is because of reduced insight into the effects of their medical condition; for others, there is a fear of losing their licence and their independence, and some people are genuinely not aware that they need to inform DVLA (College of Occupational Therapists, 2012).

Occupational therapists are now able to report concerns directly to the DVLA although it is more likely that the occupational therapist will support the person living with a long-term neurological condition to understand their legal responsibilities in the first instance (College of Occupational Therapists, 2012). Sharing confidential information with an outside agency needs to be considered carefully as occupational therapists are required to protect the person living with a long-term neurological condition's right to confidentiality (College of Occupational Therapists, 2012). However in these circumstances there is also a duty to protect the general public (College of Occupational Therapists, 2010). Occupational therapists should discuss their concerns with the person living with a long-term neurological condition and seek to obtain consent to disclose relevant information to the DVLA (College of Occupational Therapists, 2012).

Fitness to drive

Once the person living with a long-term neurological condition has informed the DVLA about their medical condition, their fitness to drive will be assessed and they may be asked to have a medical examination. A decision will then be made with the following recommendations:

- Allowed to keep a full licence
- Given a temporary licence, valid for 1–3 years
- Given a licence to drive an automatic car or one with specialist controls
- In extreme cases, refused a licence.

Driver rehabilitation

Occupational therapists support safe driving through rehabilitation of cognitive, motor and perceptual skills (CAOT, 2009). People living with a long-term neurological condition may also be encouraged to make some practical changes to the way they drive including (Rica, 2013):

- Avoiding driving in certain conditions, for example in the dark, when it is raining and at busy times of the day
- Slowing down to increase reaction time
- Taking extra care when approaching a junction or a hazard
- Taking time when moving off, making sure all surrounding areas have been checked
- Avoiding pressure from other drivers
- Planning journeys to avoid pressure

- Planning the route, including consideration of options for parking your route
- Allowing time for rests
- Feeling positive about stopping – as long as it is safe to do so!

Vehicle modification

Many modern cars have features which are designed to make them easier and safer to drive which can include the following (Rica, 2013):

- Variable power steering
- Brake assist and traction control
- Automatic or semi-automatic gear boxes
- Cruise control
- Hill start assist
- Automatic headlights and wipers
- Parking sensors and cameras.

The following accessories and adaptations can also help make it easier to drive (Rica, 2013):

- Panoramic rear-view mirrors
- Coloured stickers to mark speed on the speedometer
- Steering balls or spinners to support one-handed steering
- Adjustable seating with lumbar support
- Adjustable steering wheel position
- Automatic transmission reduces gear changes
- Brake assistance
- Hand controls
- Steering column-mounted controls
- Modified door hinges or extensions to seat runners to create more space for getting in and out of the vehicle
- Height adjustable, swivel mechanisms or replacement seats

Supporting driving cessation

If the person living with a long-term neurological condition is finding it difficult to drive or feeling concerned about their own and other's safety, they may choose to drive less or even stop driving (Rica, 2013). Driving cessation can lead to restricted community engagement (Marottoli et al., 2000), changes to identity and self-esteem (Eisenhandler, 1990) and increased depressive symptomatology (Ragland et al., 2005). Driving cessation can impact upon quality of life, participation in life roles, independence and safety (Ralston et al., 2001).

In general, driving cessation is a gradual, voluntary process (Liddle and McKenna, 2003). While a small proportion of people living with a long-term neurological condition cease driving because they have their licences revoked, most do so for reasons related to health status, advice from family and feeling uncomfortable or anxious with the driving role (Liddle and McKenna, 2003). The difficulties which contribute to driving cessation can of course create challenges to the use of alternative forms of transport such as mobility problems making it difficult to use public transport (Liddle and McKenna, 2003). This may significantly impact on social and leisure activities and participation (Liddle and McKenna, 2003). Reliance on informal carers for transport may also place additional burden and may further restrict the opportunities for engagement and participation (Liddle and McKenna, 2003).

Driving cessation therefore requires a planned and structured approach to ensure the transition to non-driver status is minimally disruptive to occupational performance, identity and self-esteem. The occupational therapist has a key role to play in supporting people living with long-term neurological conditions to prepare for this adjustment.

9.7 Caregiving

There are approximately 850 000 people in the United Kingdom looking after someone living with a long-term neurological condition (Jackson et al., 2013). The primary carers of people with a long-term neurological condition are usually a family member and mainly a spouse (Aoun et al., 2011). They spend on average between 20 and 50 hours per week caring for their family member (Jackson et al., 2013).

9.7.1 Impact on family and carers

Experiences of carers vary widely (Martinez-Martin et al., 2008; Schrag et al., 2006), with some carers adapting and coping well throughout the disease (Abendroth et al., 2012). However for others, caring for a person living with a long-term neurological condition can have a variety of negative physical, psychological, social and financial consequences for carers that may challenge their ability to continue their caring role (Greenwell et al., 2015).

Carers of people living with a long-term neurological condition can be faced with increased worry and uncertainty over their future; feelings of guilt, grief and frustration; negative changes in lifestyle, including restricted work and social activities; and a worsening financial situation, mainly through loss of earnings (Greenwell et al., 2015). The overall impact can lead to poor psychosocial outcomes including reduced quality of life, emotional and financial strain, fatigue, sleep disturbances, social isolation and an increased risk of neuropsychiatric symptoms and chronic illness (Greenwell et al., 2015).

Challenges also occur due to the sometimes unremitting commitment involved in the care of a person living with a long-term neurological condition involving responsibilities such as providing emotional support, controlling feeding and fluids, learning new strategies for communication as speech deteriorates, striving to plan ahead in a situation of constant change, managing medical equipment and increasing demands in relation to moving and handling (Birks, 2008).

Carers face daily changes as well as long-term adjustments as they worry about illness progression and the overall well-being of the family (Bromberg and Forshew, 2002; Trail et al., 2004), changes in family roles (Hughes et al., 2005; Lackey and Gates, 2001), loss of sexual relationships (Kaub-Wittemer et al., 2003; O'Connor et al., 2008), loss of a reciprocal relationship with spouse carers (Ray and Street, 2007) and, in some situations, being blamed by other family members for inadequate care (Martin and Turnbull, 2001).

9.7.2 Burden of care

Burden of care is defined as 'the extent to which the caregivers perceive their health, social life and financial status are suffering because of their caregiving experience' (Zarit et al., 1980). Recent studies of carers of people with Parkinson's have highlighted that carer age and length of time in the caregiving role are of importance, and females appear more vulnerable in their caring role than males (Morley et al., 2012). The intensity of caregiving (informal hours and years of caregiving) was shown to correlate with carer burden (Greenwell et al., 2015).

Factors which contribute to increased carer strain include the following:

- Losing the ability to walk
- Increased amount of time spent on toileting, bathing, dressing, administering medications and feeding (Chio et al., 2006)
- Respiratory and breathing difficulties (Gysels and Higginson, 2009)
- Feeling ill-prepared to cope, causing anxiety, depression and distress
- Behavioural problems (Schumacher et al., 2006).

At the end of life, as family carers lose the ability to interact with their loved ones, they may begin to struggle with meaning and feel powerless (Rabkin et al., 2006). There is increasing evidence to indicate that people with a long-term neurological condition and their family carers do not always hold the same attitudes or beliefs about care (Bolmsjo and Hermeren, 2003) or agree about treatment course or end-of-life decision-making (Trail et al., 2003). People living with a long-term neurological condition may refuse life-sustaining treatments, such as tracheostomy or assisted ventilation (Kaub-Wittemer et al., 2003) or may have an interest in hastening death, all of which can cause distress for carers (Rabkin et al., 2000). The impact of long-term neurological conditions can continue to affect families after death, despite the end to caregiving (Aoun et al., 2013). In bereavement, carers can experience lasting emotional impacts, including sadness, fear, frustration, hatred and anger, depression and, for some, hopelessness (Hebert et al., 2005).

9.7.3 Supporting carers

Occupational therapists can support carers in a number of ways by:

- Providing direct support to family carers to meet their practical and emotional needs
- Providing interventions that support the existential and spiritual concerns of people with long-term neurological conditions and their family carers

- Delivering compassionate care at the time of diagnosis and throughout the disease trajectory
- Providing practical advice and guidance on symptom management, technology and meeting personal care needs
- Open and genuine communications to share concerns and identify needs.

9.7.4 Supporting the needs of young carers

Being a young carer is much more common than perhaps thought with at least 175 000 in the United Kingdom (MS Society, 2008). Young carers help with many aspects of daily life including the following:

- Housework
- Household shopping
- Cooking
- Looking after siblings
- Looking after the person living with a long-term neurological condition
- Supporting other members of the family.

Young carers may require a different level of support due to the following reasons:

- Adjustment to the diagnosis of a family member with a long-term neurological condition
- Impact on parental relationships
- An unwillingness to 'burden' family member with their own needs
- The impact on their own occupational performance and ability to engage in meaningful occupations
- Achieving occupational balance between caring role and schoolwork
- Emotional challenges including anger and frustration, worry, guilt, jealousy, loneliness, sadness and embarrassment
- Financial pressures
- Social pressures including bullying as their family is seen as 'different' or becoming the bully as a way to vent anger and frustration (MS Society, 2008).

Occupational therapists can support young carers by:

- Talking to them and helping them to understand the medical condition
- Talking to them about their own needs
- Recognising risks factors
- Providing practical support, for example equipment or adaptations
- Promoting a healthy lifestyle including eating properly and exercise
- Providing information and support.

9.8 Psychosocial adjustment

The majority of people living with a long-term neurological condition make a positive adjustment as indicated by maintenance of a positive self-concept despite the chronic and progressive nature of their diseases (Brooks and Matson, 1982).

Psychosocial well-being reflects a position in which the person living with a long-term neurological condition perceives a state of harmony in all aspects of their life (Orem, 1985). Models of psychosocial adaptation describe three stages of reactions (Livneh, 2001) as follows:

1 Earlier reactions: (shock, anxiety and denial)
2 Intermediate reactions (depression, internalised anger and externalised anger)
3 Later reactions (acknowledgement and adjustment).

   Psychosocial adaptation involves a continuous process of adjustment which allows people to work through the initial shock and uncertainty of a diagnosis discarding both false hope and feelings of hopelessness until they can attribute meaning and purpose to living with the limitations imposed by the illness (Feldman, 1974).

   Major psychosocial adjustment most commonly occurs within the first 10 years of diagnosis with a long-term neurological condition (Brooks and Matson, 1982). Physical health status has the greatest influence on psychosocial adaptation affecting self-confidence, self-reliance and social interactions (Zeldow and Pavlou, 1984). The greater the impact of a long-term neurological condition on a person's ability to participate in everyday activities, the more likely the person is to demonstrate a lower self-concept (Brooks and Matson, 1982). Uncertainty in disease course also contributes to difficulties in adjustment (Antonak and Livneh, 1995).

Jane Duffy's story

'My journey begins when I was born in 1965, I had an older brother and we lived with my parents until I left home to train to be an occupational therapist (OT) in 1985.

The professional me

I trained as an occupational therapist in Derby in England. After I qualified in 1988, I moved to Hull in Humberside, working with adults with profound learning and physical disabilities. I moved up to Scotland after about a year and began my career in Social Services, working with people with physical disabilities and sensory impairment.

The family me

I met my future husband, when I was in second year, an Irish man, brought up in Scotland and working in Wales. Our daughter was born in August 1989. We moved to Ayrshire in 1990.

HD – The beginning

I haven't had any contact with my brother and sister-in-law for over 20 years. In early January 2012, my sister-in-law emailed me to ask if I knew of any inherited illnesses in the family history as she was concerned about my brother's health, she thought he might have Parkinson's. She had also said that my Aunt had been diagnosed with Huntington's disease (HD). There was no history of HD in the family. It was clear that my sister-in-law had not made any link between what she described as my brother's symptoms at this time, with my Aunt's illness.

On reflection, I thought that my mum may well have had HD, but she was never diagnosed with it. When she first attempted suicide, I was still doing my occupational therapist training, I all but begged her psychiatrist to look at the whole person and the whole picture, instead of lots of different medical professionals treating a singular symptom or problem.

This didn't happen and mum took her own life in 1991. It is my belief that if she had been correctly diagnosed, and got the help she needed, she would not have completed suicide when she did. I will never be able to begin to put myself in her shoes.

The genetic testing process

I decided to go through the genetic testing process. I received the results in June 2012. I can only describe the feeling on receiving this "bad" news, as like being hit with a cricket bat. This result also means that my daughter has a 50/50 chance of having the faulty gene, and she has to make decisions about whether to be tested and having children herself which none of us should ever have to make.

My daughter graduated 4 weeks after the test result – I hadn't told her the news, there was no "right time" to tell your daughter that you will develop HD, and that there is a 50% chance that I have passed that gene mutation onto her…I waited until after her birthday and then her summer holiday with her pals before I told her. I can't explain how difficult that was, or how it felt to have to tell the most precious thing in my life the news, and all that meant, for both her and me. It is the most difficult thing I have ever had to do in my life; it was the first time as a mother that I could do absolutely nothing to make things better.

Who I was then

A mother	A wife	A sister	A daughter
A relative	An OT	A colleague	A service manager
A friend	A boss	An MSc student	An employee

The diagnosis

At this time, I was having difficulties with my speech, difficulties cooking and driving, cognitive difficulties and other problems functioning at work, including concentration and excessive tiredness for several months, I was advised by medical practitioners that this was stress. In April 2013, I hit a brick wall and had to go "off sick" from my job. Following a cognitive assessment, an assessment of mood and a MRI, I was advised I was HD symptomatic on 5 August 2013. I left work on 30 September 2013 on ill-health grounds. I am making this process and this decision sound easy; you will understand that this was another hugely difficult process to go through, and the decision relating to my career was immense one for me – who would I be if I didn't have my career?

Living for each day

- Learning to manage my symptoms – accepting, accommodating, adapting and changing
- Prioritising on a daily basis
- Working to devise strategies for even the most simplest of things.
- Working through my "FINDY" (F*** I'm Not Dead Yet) list – currently learning to groom and ride horses (with a lot of support)
- Cat Protection Volunteer when I feel well enough

- Involvement in clinical research
- Planning for the future.
- There were a significant amount of practical issues that had to be addressed at this time:
- Developing my FINDY list, including my priorities for the time that I still have an acceptable quality of life.
- Financial planning: mortgage, endowment policies, life insurance, permanent health insurance, pension, debts
- Career and profession
- Legal planning: will, Power of Attorney
- Health planning: Advance statement, advance care plan, do not attempt cardiopulmonary resuscitation (DNA CPR), brain donation
- End-of-life and funeral planning
- Adaptations to ensure I don't have to move from my home.

I began to have difficulty swallowing early in 2014; eventually, I was concentrating solely on the act of swallowing rather than the pleasure of food and mealtime conversations. This, combined with a complete lack of appetite and no longer having the ability to cook, was having a significant impact on my overall well-being, and I was losing weight too quickly.

When my speech also started to deteriorate further, I couldn't pronounce specific sounds and words; I was slurring and stammering, forgetting words and using the wrong words and so on. I was referred to the speech and language therapy service. By this time, I had become insular and withdrawn; I wouldn't go out socially, I had completely lost my spark and had zero self-confidence. As an experienced allied health professional (AHP), I never realised the depth to which these kinds of issues can impact on an individual with HD.

I was facing the stark realisation that the outcome will be my inability to speak and swallow, and the likelihood of developing increasing chest infections, which will eventually lead to my death. I had already stated in my advance care plan that I do not want percutaneous endoscopic gastrostomy (PEG) intervention, but now I didn't feel ready to die. It is very easy to get subsumed by the enormity and impact of HD, but I will continue to live my life with it, rather than dying with it.

Whatever my degree of disability in the future, no matter how many different services and professionals will need to be involved in supporting me to continue to live at home, I will always be all of the things highlighted below.

Who I am now

A mother	A wife	A sister	A daughter
A relative	An OT	A colleague	A service manager
A friend	A boss	An MSc student	An employee

(Not Just) A Patient!

More importantly, I want to be an individual with a personal story which has made me who and what I am, not just another patient.

I liken having HD to skiing uphill in an "avalanche risk" area, it is difficult enough not to be subsumed by the enormity and impact of the disease; but with each significant deterioration, the avalanche pushes me back down the mountain. The only way I can get back on the "black run" is with my own team of medical and AHP professionals that I can both trust and rely on, who are knowledgeable and experienced about both this disease and recognise me as an individual person with my own priorities and not as just another patient (or CHI number) with this disease'.

9.9 Self-evaluation questions

1 What are the key elements of transition which may be experienced by people diagnosed with a long-term neurological condition?
2 How can occupational therapists support people at the time of diagnosis with a long-term neurological condition?
3 What are the key elements of rehabilitation for people with long-term neurological conditions?
4 What factors might couples need to consider when planning a family if there is a family history of a long-term neurological condition?
5 What are the key factors which impact on the ability to remain in work?
6 What are the main concerns about disclosing a long-term neurological condition to an employer?
7 How might carers of people with long-term neurological conditions be affected?
8 What are the key factors which lead to burden of care for carers of people with long-term neurological conditions?
9 How are young carers affected?
10 Which theories of psychosocial adjustment can be applied to long-term neurological conditions?

References

Abendroth M, Lutz BJ and Young ME (2012) Family carers' decision process to institutionalise persons with Parkinson's disease: a grounded theory study. International Journal of Nursing Studies, 49:445–454.

Adams J, Hayes J and Hopson B (1976) Transition: understanding and managing personal change. London: Martin Robertson.

Antonak RF and Livneh H (1995) Psychosocial adaptation to disability and its investigation among persons with multiple sclerosis. Social Science and Medicine, 40(8):1099–1108.

Aoun AM, Connors SL, Priddis L, Breen LJ and Colyer S (2011) Motor Neurone Disease family carer's experiences of caring, palliative care and bereavement: an exploratory qualitative study. Palliative Medicine, 26(6):842–850.

Aoun AM, Bentley B, Funk L, Toye C, Grande G and Stajduhar KJ (2013) A 10-year literature review of family caregiving for motor neurone disease: moving from caregiver burden studies to palliative care interventions. Palliative Medicine, 27(5):437–446. DOI:10.1177/0269216312455729.

Baldwin C and Brusco NK (2011) The effect of vocational rehabilitation on return-to-work rates post stroke: a systematic review. Topics in Stroke Rehabilitation, 18(5):562–572.

Birks C (2008) Inquiry into better support for carers. Gladesville, NSW: MND Australia.

Bolmsjo I and Hermeren G (2003) Conflicts of interest: experiences of close relatives of patients suffering from amyotrophic lateral sclerosis. Nursing Ethics, 10(2):186–197.

Bromberg M and Forshew D (2002) Comparison of instruments addressing quality of life in patients with ALS and their carers. Neurology, 58:320–322.

Brooks NA and Matson RR (1982) Social-psychological adjustment to multiple sclerosis: a longitudinal study. Social Science and Medicine, 16(24):2129–2135.

Canadian Association of Occupational Therapists (2009) CAOT Position statement: occupational therapy and driver rehabilitation. Ottawa, ON: Canadian Association of Occupational Therapists.

Chio A, Gauthier A, Vignola A, Calvo A, Ghiglione P, Cavallo E, Terreni AA and Mutani R (2006) Caregiver time use in ALS. Neurology, 67(5):902–904.

College of Occupational Therapists (2010) Code of ethics and professional conduct. London: College of Occupational Therapists.

College of Occupational Therapists (2012) Briefing 26 – service user's fitness to drive. London: College of Occupational Therapists.

Dyck I and Jongbloed L (2000) Women with multiple sclerosis and employment issues: a focus on social and institutional environments. Canadian Journal of Occupational Therapy, 67:337–346.

Eisenhandler S (1990) The asphalt identikit: old age and the driver's licence. International Journal of Aging and Human Development, 30(1):1–14.

Escorpizo R, Reneman MF, Ekholm J, Fritz J, Krupa T, Marnetoft SU, Maroun CE, Guzman JR, Suzuki Y, Stucki G and Chan CCH (2011) A conceptual definition of vocational rehabilitation based on the ICF: building a shared global model. Journal of Occupational Rehabilitation, 21(2):126–133.

Feldman DJ (1974) Chronic disabling illness: a holistic view. Journal of Chronic Disease, 27: 287–291.

Franche RL and Krause N (2002) Readiness for return to work following injury of illness: conceptualising the interpersonal impact of health care, workplace, and insurance factors. Journal of Occupational Rehabilitation, 12(4):233–256.

George LK (1993) Societal perspectives on life transitions. Annual Reviews Sociology, 19:353–373.

Greenwell K, Gray WK, van Wersch A, van Schaik P and Walker R (2015) Predictors of the psychosocial impact of being a carer of people living with Parkinson's disease: a systematic review. Parkinsonism and Related Disorders, 21:1–11.

Gutenbrunner C, Meyer T, Melvin J and Stucki G (2011) Towards a conceptual description of physical and rehabilitation medicine. Journal of Rehabilitation Medicine, 43: 769–764.

Gysels MH and Higginson IJ (2009) Caring for a person in advanced illness and suffering from breathlessness at home: threats and resources. Palliative and Supportive Care, 7(2):153–162.

Hawley C (2001) Return to driving after head injury. Journal of Neurology, Neurosurgery and Psychiatry, 70(6):761–766.

Hebert RS, Lacomis D, Easter C, Frick V and Shear MK (2005) Grief support for informal caregivers of patients with ALS: a national survey. Neurology, 64:137–138.

HMSO (2010) The Equality Act. London: The Stationery Office.

Hughes RA, Sinha A, Higginson IJ, Down K and Leigh PN (2005) Living with motor neurone disease: lives, experiences of services and suggestions for change. Health and Social Care in the Community, 13(1):64–74.

Huntington's Disease Association (2012) Huntington's disease predictive testing. Liverpool: Huntington's Disease Association.

Jackson D, McCrone P and Turner-Stokes L (2013) Costs of caring for adults with long term neurological conditions. Journal of Rehabilitation Medicine, 45(7):653–661

Johnson KL, Klasner ER, Amtmann D, Kuehn CM and Yorkston KM (2004) Medical, psychological, social and programmatic barriers to employment for people with multiple sclerosis. Journal of Rehabilitation, 70:38–49.

Kaub-Wittemer D, Steinbuchel Nv, Wasner M, Laier-Groeneveld G and Borasio GD (2003) Quality of life and psychosocial issues in ventilated patients with amyotrophic lateral sclerosis and their caregivers. Journal of Pain and Symptom Management, 26(4):890–896.

Kralik D, Brown and Koch T (2001) Women's experiences of 'being diagnosed' with a long-term illness. Journal of Advanced Nursing, 33(5):594–602.

Kralik D, Visentin K and van Loon A (2006) Transition: a literature review. Journal of Advanced Nursing, 55(3):320–329

Krause I, Kern S, Horntrich A and Ziemssen T (2013) Employment status in multiple sclerosis: impact of disease-specific and non-disease-specific factors. Multiple Sclerosis Journal, 19(13): 1792–1799.

Lackey NR and Gates MF (2001) Adults' recollections of their experiences as young caregivers of family members with chronic physical illnesses. Journal of Advanced Nursing, 34(4):320–328.

Liddle J and McKenna K (2003) Older drivers and driving cessation. British Journal of Occupational Therapy, 66(3):125–132.

Livneh H (2001) Psychosocial adaptation to chronic illness and disability: a conceptual framework. Rehabilitation Counseling Bulletin, 44(3):151–160.

Marottoli R, Mendes de Leon C, Glass T, Wiliams C, Cooney L and Berkman L (2000) Consequences of driving cessation: decreased out of home activity levels. Journal of Gerontology: Social Sciences; 55:334–340.

Martin J and Turnbull J (2001) Lasting impact in families after death from ALS. Amyotrophic Lateral Sclerosis Other Motor Neurone Disorders, 2:181–187.

Martinez-Martin P, Arroyo S, Rojo-Abuin JM, Rodriguez-Blazquez C, Frades B and de Pedro Cuesta J (2008). Burden, perceived health status and mood among caregivers of Parkinson's disease patients. Movement Disorder, 23:1673–1680.

Meleis AI, Sawyer LM, Im EO, Hilfinger Messias DK and Schumacher K (2000) Experiencing transitions: an emerging middle-range theory. Advances in Nursing Science, 23(1):12–28.

Morley D, Dummett S, Peters L, Kelly P, Hewitson P, Dawson J, Fitzpatrick R and Jenkinson C (2012) Factors influencing quality of life in caregivers of people with Parkinson's disease and implications for clinical guidelines. Parkinson's Disease, 2012:190901, DOI:10.1155/2012/190901.

Multiple Sclerosis Society (2008) MS in your life – a guide for young carers. London: Multiple Sclerosis Society.

Multiple Sclerosis Society (2010) Work and MS – for employees and employers. London: Multiple Sclerosis Society.

O'Connor EJ, McCabe MP and Firth L (2008) The impact of neurological illness on marital relationships. Journal of Sex and Marital Therapy, 34(2):115–132.

Orem DE (1985) A concept of self-care for the rehabilitation client. Rehabilitation Nursing, 10:33–36.

Parker RM, Szymanski EM and Patterson JB (2005) Rehabilitation counselling: basics and beyond, 4th Edition. Austin, TX: Pro-Ed.

Paterson BL (2001) The shifting perspectives model of chronic illness. Journal of Nursing Scholarship, 33(1):21–26.

Playford ED, Radford K, Burton C, Gibson A, Jellie B, Sweetland J and Watkins C (2011) Mapping vocational rehabilitation services for people with long term neurological conditions: summary report. London: Department of Health.

Preston JA (2009) Executive function and multiple sclerosis: implications for occupational therapy practice. PhD Thesis, Glasgow Caledonian University, Glasgow.

Preston J, Ballinger C and Gallagher H (2014) Understanding the lived experience of people with multiple sclerosis and dysexecutive syndrome. British Journal of Occupational Therapy, 77(10):484–490.

Rabkin JG, Wagner GJ and Del Bene ML (2000) Resilience and distress among amyotrophic lateral sclerosis patients and caregivers. Psychomatic Medicine, 62:271–279.

Rabkin JG, Albert SM, Tider T, Del Bene ML, O'Sullivan I, Rowland LP and Mitsumoto H (2006) Predictors and course of elective long-term mechanical ventilation: a prospective study of ALS patients. Amyotrophic Lateral Sclerosis, 7(2):86–95.

Radford K, Phillips J, Drummond A, Sach T, Walker M, Tyerman A, Haboubi N and Jones T (2013) Return to work after traumatic brain injury: cohort comparison and economic evaluation. Brain Injury, 27(5):507–520.

Ragland D, Satarinano W and MacLeod K (2005) Driving cessation increased depressive symptoms. Journal of Gerontology: Medical Sciences, 60(3):339–403.

Ralston L, Bell S, Mote J, Rainey T, Brayman S and Shotwell M (2001) Giving up the car keys: perceptions of well elders and families. Physical and Occupational Therapy in Geriatrics, 19(4):59–70.

Ray RA and Street AF (2007) Non-finite loss and emotional labour: family caregivers' experience of living with motor neurone disease. Journal of Clinical Nursing, 16(3A):35–43.

Rica (2013) Driving safely for life: a guide on keeping safe and driving for as long as possible. London: Rica.

Roessler RT (1996) The role of assessment in enhancing the vocational success of people with multiple sclerosis. Work, 6:191–201.

Roessler RT and Rumrill PD (1995) The relationship of perceived work site barriers to job mastery and job satisfaction for employed people with multiple sclerosis. Rehabilitation Counselling Bulletin, 39:2–14.

Roessler R, Fitzgerald S, Rumrill P and Koch L (2001) Determinants of employment status among people with MS. Rehabilitation Counselling Bulletin, 45:31–40.

Roessler R, Rumrill P and Fitzgerald S (2004) Predictors of employment status for people with multiple sclerosis. Rehabilitation Counselling Bulletin, 47:96–103.

Rumrill P (2009) Challenges and opportunities related to the employment of people with multiple sclerosis. Journal of Vocational Rehabilitation, 31:83–90.

Rumrill P, Hennessey M and Nissen S (2008) Employment issues and multiple sclerosis, 2nd Edition. New York: Demos.

Schrag A, Hovris A, Morley D, Quinn N and Jahanshahi M (2006) Caregiver burden in Parkinson's disease is closely associated with psychiatric symptoms, falls and disability. Parkinsonism Related Disorders, 12:35–41.

Schumacher K and Meleis A (1994) Transitions: a central concept in nursing. Journal of Nursing Scholarship, 26(2):119–127.

Schumacher K, Beck CA and Marren JM (2006) Family caregivers: caring for older adults, working with their families. American Journal of Nursing, 106(8):40–49.

Simmons R, Tribe K and McDonald E (2010) Living with multiple sclerosis: longitudinal changes in employment and the importance of symptom management. Journal of Neurology, 257:926–936.

Sinclair E, Radford K, Grant M and Terry J (2014) Developing stroke-specific vocational rehabilitation: a soft systems analysis of current service provision. Disability and Rehabilitation, 36(5):409–417.

Strober L, Christodoulou C, Benedict R, Westervelt H, Melville P, Scherl W, Weinstocj-Guttman B, Rizvi S, Goodman A and Krupp L (2012) Unemployment in multiple sclerosis: the contribution of personality and disease. Multiple Sclerosis Journal, 18(5):647–653.

Sweetland J, Riazi A, Cano SJ and Playford ED (2007) Vocational rehabilitation services for people with multiple sclerosis: what patients want from clinicians and employers. Multiple Sclerosis, 13:1183–1189.

Trail M, Nelson ND and Van JN (2003) A study comparing patients with amyotrophic lateral sclerosis and their caregivers on measures of quality of life, depression, and their attitudes toward treatment options. Journal of the Neurological Sciences, 209(1–2):79–85.

Trail M, Nelson N, Van JN, Appel SH and Lai EC (2004) Major stressors facing patients with amyotrophic lateral sclerosis (ALS): a survey to identify concerns and to compare with those of their caregivers. Amyotrophic Lateral Sclerosis Other Motor Neuron Disorders, 5(1):40–45.

Varekamp I, de Vries G, Heutink A and van Dijk F (2008) Empowering employees with chronic diseases: development of an intervention aimed at job retention and design of a randomised controlled trial. BMC Health Service Research, 8:224.

Yorkston KM, Johnson K, Klasner ER, Amtmann D, Kuehn CM and Dudgeon B (2003) Getting the work done: a qualitative study of individuals with multiple sclerosis. Disability Rehabilitation, 25:369–379.

Young AE, Roessler RT, Wasiak R, McPherson KM, van Poppel MN and Anema JR (2005) A developmental conceptualization of return to work. Journal of Occupational Rehabilitation, 15(4):557–568.

Zarit SH, Reever KE and Bach-Peterson J (1980) Relatives of the impaired elderly: correlates of feelings of burden. Gerontologist, 20:649–655.

Zeldow PB and Pavlou M (1984) Physical disability, life stress, and psychosocial adjustment in multiple sclerosis. Journal of Nervous and Mental Disease, 172(2):80–84.

Zheltoukhova K (2011) Providing support for employees with MS. Occupational Health, 63(9):24–25.

CHAPTER 10

Planning for the future

10.1 Introduction

Occupational therapy has a clear role in helping and enabling people living with long-term neurological conditions and their carers or family to plan for their future, by helping them aim to achieve their occupational goals regardless of the stage of their disease, life expectancy or disability (National End of Life Care Programme/College of Occupational Therapists, 2012). Long-term neurological conditions may result in severe impairments which reduce the client's autonomy, altering the aspirations and hopes of them and their families (Giovagnoli et al., 2009). They will, therefore, need to work out strategies with the occupational therapist to help cope with this change in occupational performance with a potentially life-limiting condition.

10.2 Disease progression

There are three key stages during disease progression when there are particular care needs of the person living with a long-term neurological condition (Oliver, 2002):

1 At diagnosis when the client and family are faced with a diagnosis that they may have little knowledge of and which may be very frightening
2 When a crisis in care occurs, such as the need to consider a new intervention, for example the use of a wheelchair, percutaneous endoscopic gastrostomy (PEG), radiologically inserted percutaneous gastrostomy (RIG), non-invasive ventilator support (NIV)
3 The terminal phase, when there is increasing deterioration and end-of-life issues are faced.

Occupational Therapy and Neurological Conditions, First Edition. Edited by Jenny Preston and Judi Edmans.
© 2016 John Wiley & Sons, Ltd. Published 2016 by John Wiley & Sons, Ltd.

Often these phases are not clearly defined and different aspects of the progression may be faced at different times for different clients (Oliver, 2002). All clients with long-term neurological conditions are different, in the disease progression itself, and how they, with their families and carers, cope with the many changes they face (Oliver, 2002). The challenge of palliative care of these clients is to ensure that all the various aspects are actively managed, involving the client and family in any decisions and changes (Oliver, 2002). The key aspects of care that need to be considered include the following (Oliver, 2002):

• Physical: particularly symptom control
• Psychological: the effects on the client
• Social: the effects on the family and carers
• Spiritual: concerns about the meaning of life and the challenges of the disease.

It is helpful to consider some of the terminology used by healthcare professionals and services available. These range from supportive care through to palliative and end-of-life care.

Supportive care: A person may receive **supportive care** for a variable amount of time even when death is not anticipated. Supportive care is defined as 'care that helps the person living with a long-term neurological condition and their family to cope with their condition and its treatment from pre-diagnosis, through the process of diagnosis and treatment, to cure, continuing illness or death and into bereavement' (National Institute for Health and Care Excellence [NICE], 2004). For example, a person living with multiple sclerosis (MS) may be receiving active treatment and may not be expected to die yet still requires supportive care.

Palliative care: Palliative care is defined as 'the active total care of patients whose disease is not responsive to curative treatment. Control of pain, of other symptoms, and of psychological, social and spiritual problems is paramount. The goal of palliative care is achievement of the best possible quality of life for patients and their families as they move towards death' (World Health Organisation, 1990). For example, the same client with MS deteriorates and active treatment does not control the disease or symptoms. As progressive deterioration and death is anticipated, the care moves from active treatment of the disease to treatment to give comfort and control symptoms, that is palliative care. On occasions, treatments that are used to actively treat disease may be used to help with symptom control as part of **palliative care**, but the aim of this treatment is to alleviate symptoms rather than aim for cure (Hanks et al., 2009).

End-of-life care: It enables the supportive and palliative care needs of both client and family to be identified and met throughout the last phase of life and into bereavement. It includes the management of pain and other symptoms and the provision of psychological, social, spiritual and practical support. End-of-life care encompasses supportive and palliative care.

It is often hard to determine exactly when a client is entering the terminal stages of life (Turner-Stokes et al., 2008). 'It seems that the way to find a philosophy that gives confidence and permits a positive approach to death and dying is to look continuously at the patients; not at their need but at their courage; not at their dependence but at their dignity' (Saunders, 1965).

This positive approach to death and dying is one that occupational therapists have embraced for many years (Pizzi and Briggs, 2004). For occupational therapists working within a rehabilitative framework however, this paradigm shift requires the development of a broader range of skills to enhance quality of life of the dying and facilitate wellness and promote healthy living until death (Pizzi and Briggs, 2004).

Occupational therapy interventions at end of life traditionally include the following (Park Lala and Kinsella, 2011):

- Addressing activities of daily living
- Providing education for energy conservation and relaxation techniques
- Addressing positioning, seating and mobility needs
- Improving comfort
- Provision of adaptive equipment
- Providing support and education for family caregivers
- Carrying out home assessments.

Case study 1

Cameron is 45 years old and was diagnosed with motor neurone disease 18 months ago. He has a wife, three children aged 6, 9 and 14, respectively, and is now wheelchair-dependent and requires hoisting for all transfers.

Whilst his immediate family is realistic and aware of his physical limitations and prognosis, his parents still hope that he will regain his strength with physiotherapy and hydrotherapy. They acknowledge that some of the equipment and adaptations has been necessary to help their son but refuse to accept much of the advice given by the occupational therapist.

The occupational therapist's approach has been to work very closely with Cameron and his wife to gently suggest certain adaptations and equipment in anticipation for his deterioration. As he has had several episodes of rapid deterioration, the occupational therapist is trying to plan ahead for the worst-case scenario whilst, at the same time, being aware that they want to keep it as a family home wherever possible. His parents find the equipment very distressing and express concerns that he will be giving in if he accepts it.

The occupational therapist uses the approach of introducing the equipment as a means of independence rather than dependence and revisits the family regularly to ensure he is managing as safely as possible. By introducing some equipment, for example wheelchair adaptations together with the physiotherapy and hydrotherapy sessions, this promotes a positive approach and helps Cameron engage with it rather than fighting against it.

With the help of the local MND, counselling and psychological help is also offered to help all parties work together to understand his condition and the reasoning behind the occupational therapists input.

10.3 The nature of occupation in death and dying

Occupation is fundamental across the lifespan yet evidence reveals important tensions that highlight various understandings of what the role of the occupational therapist at end of life entails. While the primary goal is to improve quality of life in the end-of-life experience, it can be less clear how occupation contributes to this goal (Park Lala and Kinsella, 2011). However, Jacques and Hasselkus (2004) found that occupation played a significant role in facilitating good dying experiences through engagement in occupations for the following:

- **Continuing life**: 'Doing the things that matter'. Many ordinary mundane occupations bring new meanings against the backdrop of dying. This includes the development of a newfound awareness of connectedness and an appreciation of day-to-day occupation.
- **Preparation for death**: 'Getting everything in order'. This involves taking care of finance and legal issues, giving up homes, giving gifts of furniture and belongings, planning funerals, passing down family history and reconciling with family.
- **Waiting**: 'It takes so long to die'. Waiting can be a solitary occupation, or it can occur in the company of others. For some clients, waiting can stretch into long periods of immobility.
- **Death and After-death**: 'A gentle good-bye'. A death experience perceived as peaceful is viewed positively by families and staff. Negative death experiences tend to be experiences in which the person was in unmanageable pain or was very anxious until actual death.

There is a developing role for occupational therapists in the care of people who are dying and their families to participate in their chosen occupations, within the limits of their illness and to their satisfaction (Keesing and Rosenwax, 2011). Palliative care aims to assist people who are dying to achieve a 'good death,' and it may be that engagement in occupations of the individual's choice contributes to the achievement of this (McNamara et al., 2004).

Case study 2

Christine is a 63-year-old lady with Huntington's disease, diagnosed 7 months ago. The clinical nurse specialist at her outpatient appointment carried identified the following concerns:

- Practical concerns
  - Grocery shopping
  - Preparing food
  - Bathing or dressing
  - Laundry or housework
- Loneliness or isolation
  - Hopelessness
- Spiritual concerns
  - Loss of meaning or purpose in life

- Physical concerns
  - Moving around or walking
  - Fatigue
  - Sleep problems
  - Personal appearance

Referral was made to the occupational therapist who worked with Christine and her husband to set goals which included assessing her home for equipment to assist daily living as well as advice on sleep patterns and fatigue management. A package of care was introduced to help alleviate the burden of domestic activities of daily living. Further work was carried out to explore activities which would be meaningful to her to provide purposeful activity and this was revisited regularly to make adjustments as required.

10.4 Facilitation of meaning, quality of life and well-being

As at all other stages of disease progression, occupational therapists have a key role in the facilitation of meaning, quality of life and well-being as people living with a long-term neurological condition approach the end of life. This can be achieved through the following (Pizzi & Briggs, 2004):

- Maximising functional ability
- Promoting comfort to support quality of life
- Assuring client and caregiver safety
- Helping clients redesign their lives and life goals
- Engaging clients in meaningful and productive occupational endeavours
- Psychosocial and psycho-spiritual enhancement via improvements or adaptations in function
- Providing support around physical, emotional and spiritual issues
- Enhancing the quality of life of the dying
- Facilitating wellness and promoting healthy living until death
- Promoting a positive approach to death

10.5 Spirituality

Spirituality can be defined as a personal search for meaning and purpose in life, which may or may not be related to religion (Tanyi, 2002). Spiritual suffering or pain may manifest itself within various domains of the client's experience. This may include physical pain, such as intractable pain, psychological pain, such as anxiety, depression, hopelessness, religious pain, such as crisis of faith, or social pain, such as when relationships break down. Although spiritual pain is not visible, the occupational therapist builds the rapport with the client and can recognise the hopelessness, helplessness or anguish of clients. This may manifest itself in desperation to escape their situation, have expectations which are impossible to meet, clutch at any new or even existing therapy or medications without any benefit. Strang et al. (2004) discuss existential pain as a metaphor for suffering.

Edwards et al. (2010) found that clients found the abstract concepts of spiritual and spirituality difficult to define. However, concepts of spirituality were related to stories about the whole of life, relationships with self and others, hope, meaning and purpose in life and the relationship with religion.

If spiritual or existential well-being imbues life with a sense of purpose or meaning, then it follows that a lack of purpose or meaning may lead to a disinvestment in life itself (Chochinov et al., 2002). Hope is related to meaning and purpose, which are key elements of the occupational therapy approach. Duggleby and Wright (2004) found that hope was defined in terms of hope for no more suffering, living each day, a peaceful death and hope for their families. To live with hope, palliative care clients had to transform hope, which involved acknowledging life the way it was and searching for meaning. This conceptual clarification offers insight into the potency of hopelessness as an experience that can undermine a sense that life has ongoing value or intrinsic worth. This clarity also has implications regarding therapeutic options that might engender a sense of meaning and purpose for clients expressing overwhelming hopelessness (Duggleby and Wright, 2005).

Amongst clients with life-threatening illness, sensing oneself as a burden to others is a theme related to quality of life, optimal palliative care and maintenance of dignity at the end of life (Cousineau et al., 2003).

Greater strength in spirituality may result in clients and caregivers having better quality of life (Lo Coco et al., 2005). Spirituality significantly contributes to predict quality of life in clients with progressive neurological conditions (Giovagnoli et al., 2009). Whilst quality of life has become an important indicator of outcome in many neurological conditions, there are of yet many unexplored personal variables. Outcome measures which are able to define detailed aspects such as forgiveness, ethical rules, inner independence, death and dying, and acceptance may be usefully considered by the occupational therapist. Some spiritual factors are independent from anxiety and depression and distinct spiritual facets may characterise a person independently from affects or emotions. Furthermore, they suggest that these elements contribute to the person being able to cope with life's challenges. Spiritual factors might influence a client's perception of impairments and disabilities or their coping strategies.

10.6 Therapeutic use of self

Within any therapeutic process and especially in work with terminally ill clients, the occupational therapist must have an awareness of and develop a therapeutic presence and be able to use one's 'self' in a therapeutic way (Pizzi and Briggs, 2004). Occupational therapists may not be aware of the power they inherently bring to the therapeutic encounter which begins as soon as they walk through the door (Pizzi and Briggs, 2004). The role of occupational therapist brings with it both power and incredible responsibility (Pizzi and Briggs, 2004). Relationship difficulties can occur when (Peloquin, 1993):

- The occupational therapist fails to see the personal consequences of illness or disability
- Therapeutic 'distance'
- Harmful withholdings
- Discouraging words
- Brusque behaviours
- Misuse of power.
    Positive behaviours include the following (Peloquin, 1993):
- Recognising that the occupational therapist is the most important therapeutic modality
- Be yourself in the process of treatment
- Be 'self-aware' of judgements, biases, prejudices, beliefs, values and joys that contribute to the therapy process and outcomes
- Engage in therapeutic and effective communications that foster a higher level of well-being for the dying and their loved ones
- Listening, not explaining, doing, or fixing is often the most important support the occupational therapist offers the dying
- By being fully present and listening without judgement, bearing witness to the person's struggle.

10.6.1 Therapist self-care

Occupational therapists are required to deliver the best quality of care to people who are dying in addition to promoting their own personal health. Pizzi and Briggs (2004) propose that it is difficult for occupational therapists to help the dying if they have not acknowledged their own uncomfortable fears about death. Honesty and introspection into our own mortality allows us to live with our own dying, and therefore better serve our clients (Sharp, 1996). Occupational therapists should seek the support of the multidisciplinary team to provide a forum to practice conversations about dying and for discussion of these significant issues of professional and personal growth (Pizzi and Briggs, 2004).

10.7 Advance care planning

Planning for the future incorporates planning safeguards into the type of ongoing treatment the client will have. The term 'living will' has no legal meaning but can be used to refer to either an advance decision or an advance statement. An advance decision is a decision to refuse treatment; an advance statement is any other decision about how one would like to be treated.

The process of advance care planning (ACP) is not just about old age; it concerns encouraging people to think about and describe ways to share their wishes to ensure they receive the medical care they would want, even when medical staff and family are making the decisions (AgeUK, 2014). This involves learning about the types of decisions that might need to be made, considering the decisions ahead of time and letting others know about these preferences, often by putting them into an advance statement. This is a legal document that goes into effect only if that person is incapacitated and unable to speak for themselves. This could be as the result of a chronic illness, injury or disease. Decisions that might arise could include resuscitation, ventilator use, tube feeding or intravenous fluids and the level of comfort such as managing symptoms and medication.

ACP discussions should be an ongoing process and can be adjusted as the situation changes because of new information or a change in health (National Hospice Council, 2012). As such, these discussions can be facilitated by any healthcare professional who has the necessary expertise and knowledge, particularly if they have a rapport with the individual. Occupational therapists may be involved in personal care and management of lifestyle and would, therefore, be able to have such a rapport. The healthcare professional needs to have adequate knowledge of the disease, treatment and the individual to be able to help discuss these issues and the preferences.

As with all such delicate issues, ACP needs to be introduced to the person in a timely and sensitive way and ask whether this is something that the individual wishes to explore (Department of Health, 2014a). Dedicated time needs to be set aside, an appointment made to sit undisturbed and discuss their wishes for the future. Such discussions are often fluid and dynamic and may occur over several meetings and should not be rushed, allowing the person the opportunity to participate and fully understand what is being covered. Clarity is essential and a review date, usually every 6 months, should be set to ensure that any changes in the person's function are taken into account (Samsi et al., 2011).

At the end of ACP discussions, the individual may decide to make a lasting power of attorney (LPA). This is a legal document allowing them to appoint someone as an attorney to make decisions about their property, affairs, health and welfare at a time in the future or at a time when they can no longer have the capacity to make decisions (AgeUK, 2014).

10.7.1 Lasting power of attorney

A power of attorney is a legal document which allows the named person or people to deal with the affairs (usually financial) of the person or 'donor' who has chosen them as their attorney (Department of Health, 2014b).

An ordinary power of attorney can be set up if the donor needs someone to act for them for a temporary period, for example while they are on holiday or in hospital or if they want to supervise their actions.

The most common type of power of attorney is an LPA which is drawn up while the donor still has mental capacity, to give permission for the person or people to deal with their affairs after they lose mental capacity. There are two types of LPA:

1 Property and financial affairs – which gives the attorney the authority to make decisions about the donor's financial affairs. They can do this even while the donor has mental capacity.
2 Health and welfare – which gives the attorney the authority to make decisions about the donor's personal welfare and healthcare.

In Scotland, powers of attorney are subject to different laws. Advice can be found on the Office of the Public Guardian (Scotland) website: http://www. publicguardian-scotland.gov.uk/power-of-attorney.

Enduring Powers of Attorney (EPA) were discontinued in October 2007, but EPAs that were set up prior to this date are still valid.

If the donor wishes to set up an LPA, it needs to be registered with the Office of the Public Guardian, information about which is on their website at the time of publication. This must be set up while the donor still has the mental capacity to make decisions.

If ordinary powers of attorney have been granted, for example because the person still has mental capacity but is unable to get to their bank or post office, they do not need to be registered, but the 'donor' or their solicitor will need to fill out a form making it clear what their powers are.

To set up an LPA, a form via the gov.uk website can be requested, or obtained from the Office of the Public Guardian or a solicitor. For ordinary powers of attorney, a form can be bought from a legal stationer, or a solicitor or local advice agency can help set one up. At the time of publication, there was currently a fee of £110 for registering each LPA. If the person wishes to register someone as their attorney for property and financial affairs, and for health and welfare, they must pay £220, though solicitors' fees vary.

If the donor receives benefits such as income support, income-based job-seeker's allowance or local housing allowance, they may be exempt from the registration fee. If the attorney pays to register the legal documents, costs can be reclaimed from the donor. Any expenses can be reclaimed, for example incurred as a result of being the attorney, such as postage and travel costs.

The authority of the attorney will be detailed in the legal document that is drawn up.

The attorney for property and financial affairs generally makes decisions such as selling property, paying the mortgage, investing money, paying bills and arranging property repairs. The attorney for personal welfare usually makes decisions such as what medical treatment the donor should have and where they should live.

An attorney must act in a highly ethical manner and only in the best interests of the donor. A decision can only be made for the donor if there is 'reasonable belief' that they lack mental capacity to make that particular decision. The required standards are set out in the Mental Capacity Act (Department of Health, 2005) and its related Code of Practice.

10.7.2 Capacity

It should be assumed that individuals have the capacity to make their own decisions. However, if there is an impairment or disturbance of the mind/brain which affects their ability to make a specific decision, their capacity needs to be tested. This involves whether they can understand the information, retain it, consider the benefits and burdens of the alternatives to the proposed treatment and communicate their decision. Any assessment of capacity has to be made in relation to a particular treatment choice. If the person has capacity, they can make the relevant decision.

However, if they do not, and the person does not have someone who can be consulted about their best interests, a decision-maker should be appointed. This is the person who has the responsibility to decide what is in the best interests if the person lacks capacity. This may require consultation with all the healthcare professionals involved in that person's care.

10.7.3 Safeguards

In the event that the person lacks capacity and has no other non-professional who can represent them, an independent mental capacity advocate (IMCA) will be appointed by a local authority or NHS Trust. The IMCA establishes the person's preferred method of communication and meets with them, using a variety of methods to ascertain their views. They gather all relevant information, documentation, consult with care givers and act as advocate in the individual's best interest (Department of Health, 2014c).

Care for clients should always be aimed at their best interests. This requires considering their beliefs and values, taking into account any written directives or statements made while that person had capacity and considering the views of those closest to that individual.

The Court of Protection and Court-Appointed Deputies also have the power to make decisions relating to the property, affairs, healthcare and personal welfare of adults who lack capacity. They can decide on whether an LPA is valid. Applications to the Court are made when there is uncertainty or disagreement about the care of the person lacking capacity.

There is also a set of safeguards called Mental Capacity Act Deprivation of Liberties Safeguards (MCA DoLS) for those living in care or staying in hospital who lack capacity, in which case the care home or hospital applies to the local authority for authorisation of deprivation of liberty. This may include restraint or staff exercising control in the person's best interests (Department of Health, 2014c).

10.7.4 Advance statement

If there has been an opportunity to plan ahead, they may have prepared a legally written statement, an advance statement. This documents their views, priorities and wishes about how they would like to be treated. It is not legally binding in the United Kingdom and should be kept with the medical notes both in hospital and in the community and with the LPA, described later.

10.7.5 Advance decision

The person may have prepared an advance decision to refuse treatment (ADRT) which only applies to a refusal of treatment. To avoid uncertainty over the validity, it must be in writing, be signed by the individual, a witness, include the date of birth and GP and must be dated (Department of Health, 2005). This is the only type of living will that is legally binding in England. It is vital that the latest legislation is explored relating to where the client lives as countries within the United Kingdom, as well as other countries throughout the world, differ.

An adult with mental capacity can refuse treatment for any reason, even if this might lead to their death. However, no one is able to insist that a particular medical treatment is given, if it conflicts with what the medical professionals providing the treatment conclude is in the client's best interests. This is why an advance decision can only be a refusal of treatment.

An advance decision cannot be used to ask for anything that is illegal such as euthanasia, help commit suicide, demand care the healthcare team considers inappropriate in your case. Nor can it be used to refuse the offer of food and drink by mouth, refuse the use of measures solely designed to maintain comfort such as providing appropriate pain relief, warmth or shelter or refuse basic nursing care that is essential to keep that person comfortable such as washing, bathing and mouth care.

It is important for those providing the treatment to feel confident that the individual has not changed their mind since the advance decision was made. If new or improved medical treatments are available, or personal circumstances have changed, its validity may be questioned if it was signed many years ago. It will also need to be checked on a regular basis to ensure it continues to reflect the individual's views. Therefore, a regular review is advisable, after which it is signed and dated again.

The advance decision can be cancelled at any time while the person still has capacity to do so. The cancellation does not have to be in writing and a verbal statement cancelling the decision should be respected. To avoid the risk that the relevant people do not know it has been cancelled, it is advisable to put the cancellation in writing, if possible, and to inform everyone who was aware of the decision's existence. The original document should be destroyed, or mark on it that it has been withdrawn (AgeUK, 2014).

10.7.6 Assisted dying and implications for occupational therapy

Bernat (2008) explained and compared ethical issues in neurological conditions such as brain death, coma, vegetative state and locked-in syndromes in terms of awareness, wakefulness, brainstem function and motor function, and how accurate diagnosis is required to care for these clients. This applies to all health-care professionals in their clinical treatment, so the occupational therapist must be clear about the treatment aims and objectives with good clinical reasoning to justify their interventions.

Distress about being a burden to others is a motivating factor in 41–75% clients asking for assisted dying (Ganzini et al., 2002; McGlade et al., 2000). Chochinov (2006) discussed the concept of burden to others and suggests a self-perception wherein clients no longer consider themselves worthy of dignity and respect. Sensing that they no longer have value, meaning or a purpose may result in their feeling that they have little or nothing to give back or contribute. For some clients, a sense of dignity cannot be separated from their core being or essence (Pullman, 2002).

The term 'dignity' has become highly politicised and is frequently invoked as justification for various end-of-life practices and policies. Death with dignity is used in relation to the right to assisted suicide and euthanasia (Sullivan et al., 2000).

Chochinov et al. (2002) suggested a model for all healthcare providers to include a broad range of physical, psychological, social and spiritual/existential issues that may affect individual client perceptions of dignity. This encompassed the key elements of occupational therapy and reinforces how occupational thera-pists can help clients plan for their future within the confines of palliative care.

When working with this client group, it is an important issue on which occu-pational therapists should reflect and be aware, therefore, of the implications for them both personally and professionally. Occupational therapists need to be open to the debate whilst in no way advocating or promoting their own moral, personal, cultural or religious opinions. They also need to be more involved in the philosophical and ethical aspects of death and dying as both the situation itself and the discussions surround it are unavoidable. This will all be influenced by one's own cultural, religious and spiritual beliefs and the occupational thera-pist should ask themselves what they would do if a client confided in them that they wanted to consider this.

Over the past few generations, there have been enormous cultural and social changes. The western death protocol has dissolved, and we no longer have the family support, the relationships with the family priest, for example that we would have had before. This was not unforeseen; we have known for decades that this layer of the fabric of society has been unravelling. But with an ever-increasing elderly population, advances in medical support and the increase in people living with neurological conditions, the occupational therapist is likely to be confronted by clients who wish to discuss assisted dying.

There is an increasing profile in the media and willingness to discuss the issue with celebrity support for assisted dying and the practice in Switzerland. Occupational therapists need to reflect on how they would handle this and ask themselves what they would do if a client told them they wished to consider this.

Occupational therapists develop therapeutic relationships and emotional bonds with the individuals who have progressive disease and may be nearing the end of their lives. This may be at a crisis point for the client. There are currently clear legal guidelines and ramifications of how the occupational therapist must respond, but these may change. Occupational therapists regularly carry out assessments in their work, and are likely to be involved in assessments if legislation changes so that healthcare professionals do provide help with assisted dying.

The occupational therapist is located at the junction, a synapse, where all these conflicting concerns meet. It is a critical point where hospital and community meet when the person leaves hospital. Occupational therapists already provide services, particularly equipment and support services, to clients at the end of their lives who are returning home which are often the focus for many coping strategies, physically, intellectually, emotionally, environmentally and socially, for the individual and their family and carers. Occupational therapists are more likely to find themselves having these discussions regarding clients taking control of the end of their lives.

Royeen and Crabtree (1999) stated that occupational therapists may be ethically challenged regarding assisted dying. They questioned whether the occupational therapist should try and encourage the person to achieve their optimum function despite their limitations or should the occupational therapist acknowledge the person's wish for assisted dying as all goals should be client focused and led by the client? If the role of the occupational therapist is to help and enable the client and the client has a deteriorating condition, then this goal cannot be met.

Communication

Factors known to impact on the communication skills of healthcare professionals include fears of letting go of strong emotions, upsetting the client, causing more harm than good and taking up too much time. Staff may also believe that it is not their role to discuss certain issues, or that they have inadequate skills to do so or there would be no support if one was to pursue this. Similarly, clients may have their own barriers in fearing admitting the inability to cope, believing the staff are too busy to listen and having difficulties in expressing themselves.

Communication skills start at the first assessment with the client and assessment should be an ongoing process throughout the course of a client's illness with structured assessments being undertaken at key points around the time of diagnosis, commencement of, and regularly throughout, the treatment, through to progression of the disease (NICE, 2004). Verbal and non-verbal communication including the use of personal space, touch, eye contact, facial expression, gestures and posture are all important elements. Broad open questions, focused questions, closed and leading questions can all be used and the use of listening skills, silences as well as encouragement and prompts are all developed with training and experience. Picking up cues, reflecting on what is spoken and clarification of information is important as well as summarising at key points (National Cancer Action Team, 2008).

The very act of acknowledging spiritual or existential distress appears to be a valuable intervention. This does require the healthcare professional being able to use appropriate language which both they and the client can understand. Chochinov et al. (2004) confirmed that the mainstay for clients approaching the end of life is supportive therapy, which aims to promote adaptive coping mechanisms, minimising maladaptive ones, and when possible, attenuating anxiety and fear.

The critical challenge can be developing compassionate and effective responses which are individually tailored and sensitive to a client's fluctuating and deteriorating health status (Chochinov et al., 2004).

Despite the knowledge that effective communication is an essential part of caring for clients, there is evidence that in practice communication continues to be problematic. Rather than issues of clinical competence, many complaints made by clients and their families reflect a perceived failure of effective communication (Healthcare Commission, 2007). Skills can be acquired and retained through training (Wilkinson et al., 2008).

Chochinov (2006) discussed how to achieve an approach that encompasses the psychosocial, existential and spiritual aspects of the client's experience. By having a greater understanding of the influence of issues including hopelessness, burden to others, loss of sense and dignity and loss of will to live, the healthcare professionals including occupational therapists have the opportunity to provide improved comfort and care for these clients.

Communication is recognised as one of the most important aspects of any therapeutic relationship. The fundamental qualities of communication between clinicians and their clients entail open-ended questions, clarification, effective use of silence and empathy. Occupational therapists must use their reflective practice and critical analysis to be flexible and listen to client's concerns and emotions.

Communication includes verbal and non-verbal aspects, but also providing information in the right amounts and at the optimum time. Reducing jargon to a minimum takes skill as well as how occupational therapists position themselves whilst engaging with the client.

Breaking bad news

Communication skills are essential in breaking bad news. Whilst the occupational therapist is unlikely to break bad news about prognosis or disease progression, they are likely to have discussions with the client about how they are managing functionally, whether this is likely to improve or deteriorate and how to plan for a staged decline. Fear of taking away a client's hope is a common reason for healthcare professionals not telling the client all the facts. However, this reason is based on misconceptions about hope. Acknowledging how people feel about receiving bad news gives them the opportunity to reflect on their feelings. The occupational therapist needs to assess each individual situation on its own merits and approach it calmly and gently, building up trust and allowing the client space and time to absorb the information.

Transference of hopelessness

Healthcare professionals want to be able to do something and give something to improve the situation. If this situation is a tragic one in which a person is dying, the occupational therapist feels better if they can provide an item of equipment. If this is useful and helps the client achieve improved quality of life and some independence, the clinical reasoning behind this intervention is appropriate. However, the clients and their families seldom actually want the occupational therapy equipment in their homes, reminding them of their loss of independence and function. Unless the occupational therapist follows up the equipment regularly, then the equipment may be likely to just clutter up the house and not be of use. In this case, the occupational therapist is transferring their hopelessness by providing a piece of equipment to try and make it better (Miller and Cooper, 2011). With symptoms such as fatigue and anxiety, the clinician has no tablet to give them to make it better, and the most effective approach is to give time by teaching coping strategies and techniques. These are advanced skills developed by the occupational therapist and by using these, the occupational therapist hands back the control to the client by enabling them to manage their symptoms.

The situation cannot be changed, but the rapport which the occupational therapist develops can help the client change the way they think about it.

Handling disappointment

The occupational therapist may need to deal with a client's disappointment due to different reasons as follows:
- If the disease progresses
- If the client and their families expectations are not met regarding support services in the community
- If their expectations are not met regarding adaptations or financial support.

The occupational therapist needs to acknowledge any bad news, and ask how the client wishes to continue coping, whether this is with adaptive equipment, support or coping techniques. This allows the client and family to have time to be sad, disappointed, upset or angry but know that they have the occupational therapist and rest of the team there for support.

10.8 Conclusion

Occupational therapists must share their practice with the multi-professional team to ensure all clinicians have up-to-date information about the client. This will enable good communication between all team members and ensure the best holistic treatment for clients in planning for their future with a neurological condition.

Clients and their families need to be aware of how the disease may affect them so that they can plan ahead with a will and if necessary, appoint an LPA and be encouraged to engage in ACP. This is a lengthy process which needs to be approached in a timely and sensitive manner, and will provide reassurance and comfort to the client and family in the event of deterioration so that the person's wishes have been fully discussed and understood.

Whilst death is, indeed, inevitable, the occupational therapist can help the client with a neurological condition plan for their future by assessing and treating them and their carers holistically. By establishing what they wish to do and achieve, the occupational therapist can help enable, empower and facilitate them in achieving their optimum independence. By addressing the physical, psychological, spiritual and social aspects of a client's being, the occupational therapist constantly reflects and challenges themselves on how to provide the best possible service to the client. This will continue to help occupational therapists in their clinical practice and enable them to be a vital part in the client's well-being, whatever the stage of the disease.

10.9 Self-evaluation questions

1 What are the three key stages of disease progression where particular care needs might exist?
2 What are the four aspects of care that need to be considered within palliative care?
3 Do I have a clear understanding of the differences between supportive care, palliative care and end-of-life care and how they work together?
4 What are the four main categories of occupation that facilitate a good dying experience?
5 Which factors can contribute to relationship difficulties between the client and the occupational therapist?
6 Do I have a clear idea of my own values and understanding of spirituality? How would I use these in my clinical reasoning?

7 How do I access emotional and professional support in my own practice?

8 Can I advise a client on advance care planning and signpost them to up-to-date and correct information?

9 What would I do if a client wished to discuss assisted suicide?

10 How do I ensure my communication skills are sufficiently competent to help clients plan for their future, and how can I develop these skills to an advanced level?

References

AGEUK (2014) Factsheet 72 advance decisions, advance statements and living wills. London: AGEUK.

Bernat JL (2008) Ethical issues in neurology, 3rd Edition. Philadelphia, PA: Lippincott Williams & Wilkins.

Chochinov HM (2006) Dying, dignity and new horizons in palliative end-of-life care. CA: A Cancer Journal for Clinicians, 56(2):84–103.

Chochinov HM, Hack T and McClement S (2002) Dignity in the terminally ill: an empirical model. Social Science and Medicine, 54(3):433–443.

Chochinov HM, Hack T and Hassard T (2004) Dignity and psychotherapeutic considerations in end of life care. Journal of Palliative Care, 20(3):134–142.

Cousineau N, McDowell I, Hotz S and Hebert P (2003) Measuring chronic patients' feelings of being a burden to their caregivers: development and preliminary validation of a scale. Medical Care, 41(1):110–118.

Department of Health (2005) Mental Capacity Act. London: Department of Health.

Department of Health (2014a) Planning for your future care. London: Department of Health.

Department of Health (2014b) Independent mental capacity advocate. London: Department of Health.

Department of Health (2014c) Deprivation of liberties safeguards briefing sheet. London: Department of Health.

Duggleby W and Wright K (2004) Elderly palliative care patients' description of hope-fostering strategies. International Journal of Palliative Nursing, 10(7):352–359.

Duggleby W and Wright K (2005) Transforming hope: how elderly palliative patients live with hope. Canadian Journal of Nursing Research, 37(2):70–84.

Edwards A, Pang N, Shiu V and Chan C (2010) The understanding of spirituality and the potential role of spiritual care in end-of-life and palliative care: a meta-study of qualitative research. Palliative Medicine, 24(8):753–770.

Ganzini L, Silveira MJ and Johnston WS (2002) Predictors and correlates of interest in assisted suicide in the final month of life among ALS patients in Oregon and Washington. Journal of Pain and Symptom Management, 24(3):312–317.

Giovagnoli AR, da Silva AM, Federico A and Cornelio F (2009) On the personal facets of quality of life in chronic neurological disorders. Behavioural Neurology, 21(3–4):155–163.

Hanks G, Cherny NI, Christakis NA, Fallon M, Kaasa S and Porteroy RK (2009) The oxford textbook of palliative medicine, 4th Edition. Oxford: Oxford University Press.

Healthcare Commission (2007) The views of hospital patients in England. London: Healthcare Commission.

Jacques N and Hasselkus B (2004) The nature of occupation surrounding dying and death. OTJR: Occupation, Participation and Health, 24(2):44–53.

Keesing S and Rosenwax L (2011) Is occupation missing from occupational therapy in palliative care? Australian Occupational Therapy Journal, 58:329–336.

Lo Coco G, Lo Coco D, Cicero V, Oliver A, Lo Verso G, Piccoli F and La Bella V (2005) Individual and health-related quality of life assessment in amyotrophic lateral sclerosis patients and their caregivers. Journal of Neurological Science, 238(1–2):11–17.

McGlade KJ, Slaney L, Bunting BP and Gallagher AG (2000) Voluntary Euthanasia in Northern Ireland: general practitioners' beliefs, experiences and actions. British Journal of General Practice, 50(459):794–797.

McNamara B, Rosenwax L, Holman C and Nightingale E (2004) Who receives specialist palliative care in Western Australia and who misses out? Perth: Uniprint, University of Western Australia.

Miller J and Cooper J (2011) The contribution of occupational therapy to palliative medicine. In Hanks G, Cherny NI, Christakis NA, Fallon M, Kassa S and Portenoy RK (Eds) Oxford textbook of palliative medicine. Oxford: Oxford University Press, pp. 206–213.

National Cancer Action Team (2008) Advanced communication skills. London: National Cancer Action Team.

National End of Life Care Programme/College of Occupational Therapists (2012) Route to success in end of life care – achieving quality for occupational therapy. London: College of Occupational Therapists.

National Hospice Council (2012) Planning for your future care. London: National Hospice Council.

National Institute for Health and Care Excellence (2004) Supportive and palliative care. London: Department of Health.

Oliver D (2002) Palliative care for motor neurone disease. Practical Neurology, 2:68–79.

Park Lala A and Kinsella E (2011) A phenomenological inquiry into the embodied nature of occupation at end of life. Canadian Journal of Occupational Therapy, 78(4):246–254.

Peloquin S (1993) The depersonalisation of patients: a profile gleaned from narratives. American Journal of Occupational Therapy, 47(9):830–837.

Pizzi M and Briggs R (2004) Occupational and physical therapy in hospice: the facilitation of meaning, quality of life and well-being. Topics in Geriatric Rehabilitation, 20(2):120–130.

Pullman D (2002) Human dignity and the ethics and aesthetics of pain and suffering. Theoretical Medicine Bioethics, 23(1):75–94.

Royeen M and Crabtree JL (1999) Assisted suicide and its implications for occupational therapists. Occupational Therapy International, 6(1):65–75.

Samsi K, Manthorpe J and Rapaport P (2011) As people get to know it more: experiences and expectations of the Mental Capacity Act 2005 amongst Local Information, Advice and Advocacy Services. Social Policy and Society, 10(1):41–54.

Saunders C (1965) The last stages of life. American Journal of Nursing, 65(3):70–75.

Sharp J (1996) Living our dying. New York: Hyperion.

Strang P, Strang S, Hultborn R and Arner S (2004) Existential pain – an entity, a provocation or a challenge? Journal of Pain and Symptom Management, 27(3):241–250.

Sullivan AD, Hedberg K and Fleming DW (2000) Legalized physician-assisted suicide in Oregon – the second year. The New England Journal of Medicine, 342(8):598–604.

Tanyi RA (2002) Towards clarification of the meaning of spirituality. Journal of Advanced Nursing, 39(5):500–509.

Turner-Stokes L, Sykes N and Silber E (2008) Long-term neurological conditions and management at the interface between neurology, rehabilitation and palliative care. Clinical Medicine, 8(2):186–191.

Wilkinson SM, Linsell L, Perry R and Blanchard K (2008) Effectiveness of a three-day communication skills course in changing nurses' communication skills with cancer/palliative care patients: a randomised controlled trial. Palliative Medicine, 22(4):365–375.

World Health Organisation (1990) Cancer pain relief and palliative care. Geneva: World Health Organisation.

Index

Printed and bound by CPI Group (UK) Ltd, Croydon, CR0 4YY

27/10/2024

14580372-0001

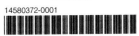